Lost in the Mirror

Lost in the Mirror

An Inside Look at
Borderline Personality Disorder

SECOND EDITION

Richard A. Moskovitz, M.D.

TAYLOR TRADE PUBLISHING
Lanham • New York • Oxford

The author gratefully thanks the following for permission to reprint previously published material:

Peter Alsop for lyrics from "Look at the Ceiling" by Peter Alsop, taken from the recording *Uniforms*. Copyright © 1981 by Moose School Music.

American Psychiatric Association for an excerpt from *Diagnostic and Statistical Manual of Mental Disorders, Fourth Edition*. Copyright © 1994 by the American Psychiatric Association.

Bantam Doubleday Dell for permission to reprint lines from *The Velveteen Rabbit* by Margery Williams.

Chrysalis Music Group for lyrics from "Hell is for Children" by Pat Benatar, Neil Geraldo, and Roger Capps. Copyright © 1980 by Chrysalis Music/Big Tooth Music/Neil Geraldo/ Muscletone Music (Ascap). International copyright secured. All rights reserved.

Houghton Mifflin Company for permission to reprint material from *Words for Dr. Y* by Anne Sexton, edited by Linda Gray Sexton. Copyright © 1978 by Linda Gray Sexton and Loring Conant, executors of the will of Anne Sexton. All rights reserved.

PolyGram Music Publishing for permission to reprint lyrics from "Candle in the Wind" by Elton John and Bernie Taupin. Copyright © 1973 Dick James Music, Ltd. All rights reserved.

William Morris Agency, Inc. for permission to reprint a line from *Gone with the Wind* by Margaret Mitchell. Copyright © 1936 by Margaret Mitchell.

Published by Taylor Trade Publishing
An Imprint of the Rowman & Littlefield Publishing Group
4501 Forbes Blvd., Suite 200
Lanham, Maryland 20706

Distributed by National Book Network

Library of Congress Cataloging-in-Publication Data
Moskovitz, Richard A.
    Lost in the mirror : an inside look at borderline personality disorder / Richard A. Moskovitz.—2nd ed.
        p.   cm.
    Includes bibliographical references and index.
    ISBN 0-87833-266-9 (pbk.)
    1. Borderline personality disorder—Popular works. I. Title.

RC569.5.B67 M67 2001
616.85'85—dc21   00-053619

Printed in the United States of America

To Betty

A gifted nurse whose compassion and serenity soothed many troubled lives.

Your friends never knew the pain held deep within your own heart.

We will miss you.

Contents

Foreword

It is a great pleasure and honor to write the foreword for this impressive work, *Lost in the Mirror*. Dr. Moskovitz is to be commended for producing this very readable book on such an intense psychiatric problem.

Through his many years' practice of psychiatry, he writes with understanding and sympathy for the thought-provoking problems of the patient. He approaches the subject with knowledge and sensitivity and leads his reader, professional and layman alike, to another level of discovery. This writing brings new insight and comprehension to concepts introduced in previous studies by other physicians and researchers. It helps one to rediscover the human significance of mental illness, conveying the desperate emptiness felt by the borderline patient while at the same time illuminating and broadening our understanding of a disorder that has already undergone intense scrutiny. Dr. Moskovitz offers both an educational source of information as well as a moving walk in another's shoes.

I have great respect for the pride and responsibility Dr. Moskovitz has invested in this work. Over the years I have discovered that people need emotional freedom for their life's journey. A personality disorder can interfere with one's ability to enjoy the true gift of living, often resulting in a nightmare of false beliefs and painful concentration on weaknesses without recognition of strengths. Through the professional attitudes and capable therapy of physicians like Dr. Moskovitz, these rigid patterns are diminished, allowing the emergence of a whole person with renewed human spirit and purpose.

This book is a valuable resource for all who seek to recognize the pain of mental illness. I believe that reviewers and readers alike will embrace this new energy and will praise this scholarly contribution.

CHRIS COSTNER SIZEMORE
Ocala, Florida, 1996
author of *The Final Face of Eve,*
I'm Eve, and *A Mind of My Own*

Preface to the First Edition

This book is written in response to years of grappling with the treatment of patients with Borderline Personality Disorder (BPD). BPD describes a complex of symptoms and behaviors that share characteristics with, or border upon, other well-defined psychiatric problems such as schizophrenia and depression. Since the term was originally coined, its own characteristics have been better defined and its distinction from other disorders better appreciated. The term "borderline" therefore refers to the derivation of the diagnosis, not to a quality of an individual.

People with BPD have been among the most engaging as well as the most provocative of my patients. They have also been among my riskiest patients because in their struggle to be alive they often tempt death. Their treatment has been ridden with crises, challenges, and opportunities for both patient and therapist to learn. My patients have taught me much about what it feels like to be them.

Despite the fact that an estimated one in ten adult women and a smaller number of men suffer from BPD, the disorder is still little known to the general public and poorly understood even by many of the professionals who treat it. As many as one in four patients in psychiatric treatment may have BPD. This still accounts for only a small fraction of people with the disorder. Even those who do find their way into treatment are often inadequately diagnosed. Their symptoms then fail to respond to treatments for anxiety, depression, bulimia, or whatever else has been identified as the problem. They may, at that point, leave treatment.

Failure to recognize BPD often results from limited information about the patient. Key symptoms, such as self-mutilation, may be withheld from the therapist out of embarrassment. The current emphasis on cost-efficient, short-term treatments also creates a tendency for some therapists to look for simple problems that can be solved quickly, perhaps with medication.

Until recently, BPD was a diagnosis that hospital staff and mental health professionals whispered behind closed doors. The diagnosis has been tainted with negativity because of the turmoil these patients bring to the treatment setting. They test our limits and probe deeply at our inadequacies.

During my years of teaching medical and psychiatry students, I have seen powerful emotional reactions to people with BPD. Some trainees become deeply entangled with such patients and develop fantasies of rescuing them from their suffering. Others find themselves suddenly involved with their patients in intense, often hostile power struggles.

The incomplete understanding of BPD shared by many providers of treatment, particularly in inpatient settings, often undermines the alliance that should develop between patient and provider to solve problems together. Any secrecy about diagnosis further undermines treatment.

For years I participated in keeping the secret. BPD was a

complex concept that seemed too difficult for patients to understand. As my own understanding of the disorder grew, primarily through experiences with patients, I began to talk more openly with my borderline patients about their diagnosis. I was surprised by their reactions.

The most striking response to this disclosure was relief. Patients expressed relief at having, at last, a comprehensive framework for understanding their suffering. They also expressed relief at discovering that they were not alone and that feelings and behaviors that made them feel "crazy" were shared by many others. Some patients disclosed new details of their personal histories once they appreciated their relevance and felt permitted to talk about them. A few patients experienced prompt improvement in symptoms and relief from suffering. Others engaged more energetically in treatment and became better able to weather the obstacles to the treatment process.

These experiences with patients stimulated the idea for this book. I became aware of the need for clear information about BPD, not only for patients but for other sufferers who have not yet found help. I became aware, too, of the need for a book that would help professionals who treat these patients understand what it feels like to be borderline.

Lost in the Mirror is written for those who have been touched by BPD. Most of us have likely had at least one encounter with someone with BPD, as it afflicts so many people. But most importantly, this book is for patients, their families, friends, lovers, and employers. It is also intended for the curious among the general public who wish to broaden their understanding of the human condition.

Lost in the Mirror is drawn to a great extent from my conversations with patients. Many of the images first occurred to me as I struggled to understand each patient's experiences and feelings. Many of the words were first spoken in actual therapeutic encounters. I have worked to preserve in the writing the atmosphere of those encounters.

This book is also a celebration of growth and of the human

potential to learn from pain. One of my early patients, as she neared the end of therapy and had become aware of the range and depth of her feelings, brought me a copy of *The Velveteen Rabbit* by Margery Williams and read me the passage quoted at the beginning of Chapter 20 in this book. Being alive, she was telling me, means being immersed in a world rich in relationships and feelings. Being Real means risking the pain that intimacy can bring and believing in yourself, flaws and all, even when faced with criticism or rejection. I am grateful to her for the message that the journey through the storm can be weathered and that identity lies at its end.

RICHARD A. MOSKOVITZ, M.D.
August 1996

Preface to the Second Edition

Since the publication of the first edition of *Lost in the Mirror*, important changes have occurred in how information is shared, in the practice of psychiatry, and in me. These changes have inspired me to write this new edition.

The Internet has become a fertile source of information on every conceivable subject. The public is better informed than at any other time in history; few secrets remain. Between the Internet and the media, many people have become acquainted with Borderline Personality Disorder. For those who would like to understand it well there are many resources, including several valuable new books and a number of web sites that provide extensive information and an opportunity for dialogue. Over the last several years, I have become well acquainted with the webmasters of several ambitious sites, which has helped me to understand better what others want to know about BPD and its treatment.

There have been significant advances over the past decade in both biological psychiatry and the practice of psychotherapy. New generations of drugs have been developed, many of which work better, faster, and with fewer side effects than their predecessors. Psychiatrists have become more adept at combining medications and blending their effects in order to bring more complete relief of symptoms. The most recent advances in the pharmacotherapy of BPD-related symptoms have been incorporated into the new Chapter 15.

The demands of managed care for briefer and more effective treatments have been partly responsible for spawning innovative forms of psychotherapy to address specific symptoms and disorders. At the same time, opportunities for getting long-term intensive inpatient therapy have become scarce as financial pressures have driven program after program out of business.

While in the first edition, I focused on the dynamics of the psychotherapeutic relationship that underlies all good treatment, in this edition I have elaborated on the kinds of psychotherapy available and how they are practiced. I have provided particularly detailed accounts of two innovative therapies, Eye Movement Desensitization and Reprocessing (EMDR) and Dialectical Behavior Therapy (DBT). EMDR, a technique for neutralizing the emotional impact of traumatic events, has infused my own practice of psychotherapy with new vitality and has expanded my understanding of the connections between past experiences and current emotions and behavior. DBT, a comprehensive treatment approach designed specifically for patients with BPD, has been a fascinating area of study that has only begun to influence my personal practice.

For those of you who are new to *Lost in the Mirror*, I hope to allow you a glimpse of what it feels like to live with this painful condition. For those who have returned to learn more, I invite you to explore the most recent innovations in pharmacological and psychotherapeutic treatments and to plumb the rich resources now available for continuing your education about Borderline Personality Disorder.

RICHARD A. MOSKOVITZ, M.D.
September 2000

1

Dear Reader

Only connect the prose and the passion, and both will be exalted, and human love will be seen at its height. Live in fragments no longer. Only connect, and the beast and the monk, robbed of the isolation that is life to either, will die.

THE LONGEST JOURNEY
E. M. FORSTER

If you are a person with Borderline Personality Disorder, this book is written especially for you. If you have spent much of your life unhappy or afraid, unable to sustain long-lasting, satisfying relationships, and have repeatedly engaged in self-defeating or injurious, impulsive behaviors, or even attempted suicide, you may well be borderline and in need of treatment.

You have been among the most gratifying and most frustrating of my patients. You have provided both the sweetest successes and the most bitter failures of my years as a psychotherapist, for you have brought to the therapeutic arena the full fury and poignancy of years of emotional turmoil. From each one of you, I have learned some valuable lessons that have, hopefully, enhanced my work with those who have followed.

You are accustomed to dealing with the world through impressions rather than ideas. When you hear a song, you listen to the music, not the words. With this book, I hope to create a living picture of your experience in the world of relationships and feelings. I have developed this picture like a painting, in layers, in keeping with your intuitive learning style. I hope the resulting images will be sufficiently vibrant and dimensional to convey to others in your life what it feels like to be you.

For years, we have kept your diagnosis secret from you for fear that you would be wounded and flee. By keeping secrets, we have promoted misunderstandings and misalliances, both with you and among those involved in your treatment. We also may have inadvertently reenacted some of the same family dynamics that have caused you pain for years, for family secrets are a way of life for most people with BPD.

This book is intended to let you in on the secret. With a clear understanding of what it means to be borderline, you may be better able to understand and predict some of your emotional reactions and behaviors. This may help you to weather the pain and continue to heal. It is my hope that the understanding that comes from this book will enable you to talk honestly about your feelings with your therapist and with other important people in your life. There will be times when this knowledge is available and useful to you, and other times when the feelings you experience are so powerful that they prevent you from remembering or using what you have learned.

This book is also intended to show you how healing occurs. Emotional pain is most difficult to bear when its origins are obscure. Many of the symptoms that you experience result from your inability to connect the memories from your past to create a cohesive and sensible story of your life. Some of these memories have been suppressed in order to protect you from being overwhelmed by particularly painful experiences. The protection, unfortunately, is incomplete and requires considerable mental energy to sustain.

Your scattered memories resemble the shards or fragments of pottery that an archeologist unearths at a dig. Each fragment provides only a hint of the form and function of the whole vessel. The fragments of one vessel may even be found interspersed among the pieces of many others, so that they must be sorted one from another before each can be reassembled.

The work of healing is like finding, sorting, and putting together the pieces of an ancient pot. The work is often tedious, and some of the slivers may be sharp and dangerous. The result, if you are patient, is a beautiful object, elegant in form and function, and eloquent in the tale it tells of its creation. If put together carefully, it will also be watertight and can be filled up with good things.

The story of Sara, which threads throughout the book at the end of each chapter, illustrates the healing process in therapy. Sara is a composite of my experiences with a number of my patients. She epitomizes both the agony and triumph that patient and therapist may experience during treatment. As you follow Sara's story, you may share in the excitement of discovering and fitting together the pieces and watching the vessel take form.

Be patient with yourself and give yourself time. If you are willing to examine your own feelings and behavior, you will gain knowledge that will enable you to be more in control of your personal history.

2

Candles in the Wind

You lived your life like a candle in the wind, never knowing who to cling to when the rain sets in.
"Candle in the Wind"
Elton John, Bernie Taupin

If you are borderline, you may experience your life as fragile and flickering, lacking in substance and permanence. You may, at times, burn brightly and intensely with emotion and, at other times, feel empty and bored. You may dart wildly about, following your impulses in a frantic effort to soothe the pain inside and create a shred of identity.

To be borderline is to have little sense of who you are or what turns you on. At its extreme, it may mean having to turn to others for cues in order to know when to eat or drink, work or rest, or even laugh or cry. It may mean intensely embracing a person, idea, or thing one day, and having no use at all for it the next. This lack of a constant picture of one's self, one's values, or one's passions is at the heart of the borderline personality. Imagine floating randomly through space without any sense of up or down and without a map to show you either your origin or your destination. To be borderline means to lack grounding emotionally and to exist from moment to moment without any sense of continuity, predictability, or meaning. Life is experienced in fragments, more like a series of snapshots than a moving picture. It is a series of discrete points of experience that fail to flow together smoothly or to create an integrated whole.

This discontinuity of experience is accompanied by a disturbing fragmentation of emotions. Feelings may vary drastically from moment to moment in quality and intensity. If you are borderline, you may alternate between being flooded with emotion and being numb to all feeling. Like a radio that has only an "on" and "off" control with the volume stuck at maximum, emotions may vary from total silence to blaring shrillness. This discontinuity of feeling is magnified by an amnesia for emotions. Whatever *feeling-state* predominates at the moment seems to last forever, and you can scarcely recall ever feeling differently. Emotional pain then becomes excruciating because it seems endless. You are unable to tap past experience and to appreciate that pain is temporary and can be survived.

When applied to relationships, this peculiar disturbance of memory means that our last encounter may be recalled as the whole of our relationship. If we last parted on an angry note, then I may be remembered as a scurrilous villain and you may wish bitterly for revenge. If we parted on more pleasing terms, then I may be remembered as an unfailing hero and you may be consumed with longing for our reunion.

With this intensely black-and-white quality of feelings, disappointment often turns to rage, which may be directed at others in fits of temper or physical attacks. Rage may also be turned against the self in the form of suicidal threats or behavior or deliberate self-injury. While self-mutilation is perhaps the most striking and shocking symptom of BPD, it is not always present. When present, it is strongly suggestive of BPD.

If you are borderline, feelings may sometimes become so intense that they distort your perception of reality. At such times you may imagine yourself deliberately persecuted by those who have merely let you down. You may even at times hear voices that tell you how to act or think.

Developing a stable sense of self depends upon being able to carry with you the memories of good relationships, memories that remain valid regardless of what is going on at the moment. If you are borderline, you have been unable to create such emotional memories, and your sense of personal value depends entirely upon what is happening in your relationships today. When you lose a relationship, you lose the inner sense of goodness that accompanied it. Since abandonment brings with it emptiness, you avoid it at all costs.

If you are borderline, you may resort to a variety of desperate, impulsive behaviors as a quick fix for painful, seemingly endless emotions, such as loneliness and anger. These behaviors may include using alcohol or other mind-altering drugs, binge eating, or engaging in impulsive sexual encounters, shopping sprees, shoplifting, and other behaviors that are self-destructive and result in additional emotional pain. At such times, the intensity of your anger may drive away those very individuals who are most capable of giving you comfort.

Elton John's characterization of Marilyn Monroe as a candle in the wind captures the essence of the borderline personality. She is an elusive character lacking in identity, overwhelmed by a barrage of painful emotions, consumed by hunger for love and acceptance, and careening from relationship to relationship and impulse to impulse in a desperate attempt to control these feelings.

If you are borderline, your desperate search for substance and meaning can end with treatment. With the help of a therapist, you can learn to curb impulses and tolerate painful emotions long enough to explore their origins. An infant, as the next chapter explains, learns to protect itself from painful emotions, which can lead to symptoms that persist into adulthood. You can learn how your fragmented world is like that of an infant who experiences the world from moment to moment and who cannot connect memories into a coherent whole. Most importantly, through your relationship with your therapist you can learn that caring can survive disappointment. As your capacity to trust in others grows, so will you learn to trust yourself. Then the winds will subside and the flame will burn clear and bright.

Diagnostic Criteria for Borderline Personality Disorder

The *Diagnostic and Statistical Manual of Mental Disorders*, fourth edition (DSM-IV), published by the American Psychiatric Association defines BPD in terms of a menu of symptoms. Because only five of nine listed symptoms are required to make the diagnosis, there is theoretically the possibility of including people with vastly different symptom complexes and little resemblance to one another. Fortunately there are unifying principles in BPD, such as the fragmentation of experience, that tie together all the symptoms and mitigate the potential diversity.

In the following presentation of the DSM-IV diagnostic criteria, I have rearranged the order to identify clusters of symptoms that belong together conceptually. These are grouped under subheadings that I have added. The identity cluster, listed first, is the most subjective and difficult to identify, but expresses the essence of BPD. The behavior cluster, listed last, is the most critical both because it contains hallmark symptoms that most easily identify people with BPD and because these symptoms most threaten patients' lives, health, and capacity to undergo treatment effectively.

According to the DSM-IV, BPD is a pervasive pattern of instability of interpersonal relationships, self-image, affects (emotions), and control over impulses beginning by early adulthood and present in a variety of contexts, as indicated by at least five of the following:

Disturbed Identity

1. Identity disturbance: self-image or sense of self persistently

and markedly disturbed, distorted, or unstable.

2. Chronic feelings of emptiness.

3. Frantic efforts to avoid real or imagined abandonment.

Disturbed Mood

4. Affective (emotional) instability due to a marked reactivity of mood. Intense, episodic dysphoria (depressed mood), irritability, or anxiety usually lasting a few hours and only rarely more than a few days.

5. A pattern of unstable and intense interpersonal relationships characterized by alternating between extremes of idealization and devaluation.

6. Inappropriate, intense anger or lack of control of anger, e.g.
   • frequent displays of temper
   • constant anger
   • recurrent physical fights

Disturbed Perception

7. Transient, stress-related paranoid ideation (feelings of persecution) or severe dissociative symptoms (discontinuity of experience, see chapter 4).

Disturbed Behavior

8. Impulsiveness in at least two areas that are potentially self-damaging:
   • spending
   • sex
   • substance abuse
   • reckless driving
   • binge eating

9. • recurrent suicidal behavior, gestures, or threats
   • self-mutilating behavior

*S*ara was thirty-one years old when we first met in her hospital room. She was an attractive woman, whose round face
and sad brown eyes were framed in ringlets of auburn hair.
She wore a low-cut green satin nightgown, more suitable for a
bedroom than a hospital room, forcing me to keep my gaze level
to respect her modesty. Her left leg was encased in a brand new
fiberglass cast from just below the knee.

Sara's orthopedic surgeon had requested the consultation
because her injury did not fit her account of the accident as she
explained it. She had been in a hurry, she said, and had closed
her car door too quickly, catching her ankle between the door
frame and the door.

The inner prominence of her ankle was fractured, but there
was no evidence of trauma to the outside of the ankle. "What's
more," the surgeon went on, "her right ankle is also badly
bruised." He suspected she had been abused, perhaps by her husband. The right ankle was bruised, but only over the outer prominence. There were also faint, horizontal linear scars over the
inner surfaces of both forearms, old injuries in a pattern that is
typically self-inflicted.

Sara was bright and engaging, a former advertising writer
and mother of two daughters: Lisa, six, and Megan, four. She had
worked until just before the birth of her younger child, when she
retired in order to care for the children full-time.

Soon after Lisa turned four, Sara had suddenly become fearful
and despondent. Within two weeks of her abrupt mood change,
she had taken an overdose of sleeping pills and was hospitalized
for psychiatric treatment. She resented the doctor and her husband for making her stay in the hospital and, early in treatment,
had made superficial cuts up and down both arms with the metal
tab from a soda can.

Sara was treated with Pamelor, an antidepressant drug, and
soon began to feel better. She was able to sleep through the
night. She looked forward to being back with the children, and
her resentment toward her husband dissipated. She no longer
wanted to die or to hurt herself. She stayed on the medication

for six weeks after discharge from the hospital, but she soon stopped keeping her appointments with the psychiatrist and ran out of medication.

Six months later, Sara had her first panic attack. It came out of the blue, late in the evening while she undressed for bed. She was in a cold sweat. Her heart pounded and her ears rang. For a few moments, her room no longer looked familiar and she had a strong urge to run away. She was overwhelmed with dread. Then it was over as mysteriously as it had begun.

When she asked her family doctor for something for anxiety, she was prescribed Valium. Over the next year, the panic attacks became more frequent, occurring almost always at night. Her Valium use increased from three tablets daily to eight to ten tablets. By the time we met, she was also drinking four to five glasses of wine each day.

As we talked, Sara's charming and seductive manner gave way to tears, then anger. She was angry at her husband, an emergency rescue worker, for trying to control her behavior. They had had numerous recent arguments about her drinking and drug use. She was also angry at herself for having recently gained fifteen pounds and she imagined herself horribly obese.

Sara also described frightening, vivid fantasies of terrible things happening to her children. She imagined them getting run over by cars or caught in a fire. She began to fear that she would somehow bring them to harm. Most of the time she watched over them vigilantly. But sometimes her husband came home to find her lost in thought or passed out while the children played unsupervised.

"I thought I had everything I ever wanted," Sara lamented, "but now all I feel is empty. I don't have any idea what's important anymore." She described waves of boredom followed by tension mounting to such intensity that she could only dispel it by causing herself physical pain. So she began hitting her ankles with the hammer, just enough to hurt. This time she had underestimated the force of the blows.

3

When She Is Good

There was a little girl
Who had a little curl
Right in the front of her forehead.
When she was good
She was very, very good.
And when she was bad
She was horrid!

"THERE WAS A LITTLE GIRL"
HENRY WADSWORTH LONGFELLOW

Unbridled rage can be terrifying. In the early weeks of life, we are unable to distinguish the pictures in our minds from what is real. To an infant, wishes are events. The rage and vengeful fantasy that accompany frustration threaten—in the infant's mind—to destroy the very person who is most crucial to security and survival.

The infant handles this terrifying anger by dividing its world neatly into good and evil. It has a good mother who feeds it when hungry and meets all of its needs unfailingly. And it has a bad mother who frustrates, ignores its cries of distress, and can be destroyed in fantasy without consequence, while the good mother remains veiled in safety.

This defensive fiction is called splitting. It is a natural outgrowth of the discontinuity of the infant's experience. While splitting normally diminishes as a child matures, it is not confined to infancy.

Splitting may serve a particularly useful function when a crucial love object, such as a parent, severely violates trust, as occurs with physical or sexual abuse. Even an abusive parent may at times be loving and nurturing and may remain crucial to the child's survival. Splitting enables the child to accept the "good parent's" love without it being tainted by something heinous.

Normally, as a child learns that people and things can last from moment to moment, the images of the good mother and the bad mother slowly merge into a consistent figure who can fundamentally be trusted to protect and provide. This image can stand up to occasional barrages of disappointment and rage, and as love forms, splitting is left behind.

If you are borderline, you may never have acquired that basic trust in a loving caretaker. Or, once having learned to trust, you may have been so betrayed that you have had to retreat to a world of discontinuity, peopled by caricatures. Your world is split into good and evil, into the stuff of which fairy tales are made—fairy godmothers and evil stepmothers, malevolent witches and rescuing princes, and very ugly frogs that suddenly transform into handsome princes.

If you are borderline, you may put me on a pedestal today and topple me tomorrow when I inevitably fail to meet your lofty expectations. You may appoint me your hero to do battle with those you have judged to be villains, or you may appoint others to do battle with me.

If you are borderline, you are likely also to split your perception of yourself. You may strive valiantly for perfection and feel, at times, that you have achieved it, only to condemn yourself when the smallest flaw appears.

When you are good, you may feel entitled to special treatment and live outside the rules made for others. You may feel entitled to take whatever you wish and to have everything good all to yourself.

When you are bad, you may feel entitled to nothing. You may feel responsible for all that is evil and expect punishment. If punishment does not come, you may invite it from others or inflict it yourself.

This paradox in attitudes may be particularly confusing to family or friends, who at one moment experience you as arrogant, demanding, and entitled, and the next as contrite, self-negating, and even suicidal.

Splitting prevents you from developing an enduring image of yourself and others and is partly behind your elusive sense of identity. Splitting is like an archeologist trying to imagine the form of a vessel by considering only one small, mineral-encrusted fragment at a time, never considering their relationship to one another.

Splitting is a defense intended to protect, but it is also a treacherous force that can destroy relationships and sabotage treatment.

Andrea was a twenty-five-year-old woman who had entered treatment to deal with her drastic mood swings and suicidal impulses. My early efforts to stabilize her moods with medication were in vain. She would arrive at my office one day full of venom for my failure to help her and another day full of gratitude for my efforts.

In time, the good days outweighed the bad, and Andrea accepted my efforts to care, showering me in return with symbolic gifts. She entertained me with her special wit and creativity, brought me meaningful cartoons (a passion of mine that she had come to know), and invested me with an aura of a special hue and quality that implied trust.

After many months of treatment, I prepared her, weeks in advance, for a ten-day vacation. I saw her several days before my departure and provided some details of my travel plans, which included an early-morning flight. Late in the evening prior to my flight, Andrea's sister called to report that Andrea had taken an overdose of medication I had prescribed. I instructed her on getting emergency medical treatment.

Enraged, Andrea called me at midnight from the emergency room and demanded that I come immediately to the hospital to attend her. When I explained that I would not change my plans and had provided for others to care for her in my absence, she fired me as her doctor. My aura had vanished.

Despite my assessment that I had done everything reasonable to attend to her needs, I could not help feeling shaken, guilty, and sad to lose this charming and colorful patient who had given me her trust.

If you are borderline, you most likely have powerful effects on other people's feelings and behavior. Your tumultuous emotions and dramatic, often provocative behaviors are sure to elicit strong reactions in others. Your environment often becomes a theater for playing out inner conflicts. Other people may become screens onto which you project feelings as if you are thinking, "Someone here is angry. It can't be me, so it must be you."

Sometimes the other people in your world fit into the roles that you have scripted for them. They may even feel the projected emotions. You may then sit back and watch your feelings being played out safely outside of yourself. You may vicariously enjoy watching others act out your fantasies, identifying with them at a distance.

Ellen was a nineteen-year-old woman who was involuntarily committed to a psychiatric hospital following a suicide attempt. Because she had felt so out of control, she was grateful for the security that I and the hospital provided. At the same time, she resented me for confining and controlling her.

During the early days of her stay, Ellen came repeatedly to me with complaints of slights at the hands of the nursing staff. She seemed so helpless and wounded that I became her willing champion, arguing for an unearned privilege here and a bend in the rules there. The nurses became frustrated with my meddling and its effects on their attempts to provide consistency and structure. The head nurse finally read me the riot act. The nurse had unwittingly acted out Ellen's wish to retaliate against me, and Ellen was left to console me in the wake of the nurse's harsh words.

The above example illustrates projective identification, a key borderline defense mechanism. Instead of expressing her anger toward me, Ellen enlisted me as an ally, and identified the nurses as the enemy. Through her successful manipulation of my behavior, Ellen's wish to retaliate against me was projected onto the staff and the projected feelings were acted out by the head nurse, while Ellen secretly savored my defeat from the sidelines.

Projective identification also means that other people believe the image that is cast upon them. Andrea, for example, believed that I was a horrible, heartless person for abandoning her at her hour of need; at the moment, so did I.

Emotional defenses protect us from experiencing uncomfortable feelings, such as shame, rage, and guilt, or from owning up to forbidden wishes that risk punishment or retaliation. Borderline defenses such as splitting, projection, and projective identification protect by maintaining distance from a living world in which real people can form lasting bonds with one another. Dissociation, another key borderline defense, is explored in the next chapter.

If you are borderline, your black-and-white thinking will probably influence your reaction to this book. You may love it and accept the entire contents uncritically, or you may hate it and reject it summarily. Most likely your reactions will be intense and will change as you read. If your initial reaction is positive, you may find something offensive later on and feel betrayed. If your first response is to throw it across the room, but you read on, you may find something of value later on that makes the reading feel worthwhile.

Your feelings about yourself as you read may reach similar extremes. Knowing that someone understands your experience may be reassuring and may help you justify your emotions. Or you may condemn yourself as you label some of your behaviors and feelings "horrid," like the girl in the poem.

While these black-and-white reactions cannot be avoided entirely, they can be modified so as not to interfere too much with your understanding. Keeping a journal is a helpful tool for reading effectively, particularly if you focus on self-affirming statements as you journal. Exploring the concepts in the book with a supportive partner may help you decide how these new ideas apply to you. If you are in therapy, this book may be a helpful companion to treatment.

Finally, reading this book can be painful. Your persistent effort to understand despite the pain is heroic and deserves affirmation.

*S*ara's earliest memories began when she was nine. She remembered a vacation at the beach when her daddy taught her to body surf. She recalled feeling his strong arms pulling her from the water after the wave had engulfed her and washed her ashore. He was her hero, and she was his shadow.

As she grew older, he took pride in all of her achievements. She was an honor student and a competitive swimmer. By the time she finished high school, she was also an accomplished graphics artist and had won statewide competitions. Her daddy never missed a swim meet or an art show.

Sara's mother was a soft-spoken, slender woman who dressed inconspicuously. She cared well for her children, but stayed always in the background of Sara's memories. She was a concerned onlooker, but barely participated in the life of the family. In its spiritual life, however, she was the leader, gathering her little family each evening after supper for a reading from the Bible. It seemed as if she sprang to life for a few minutes each evening and then faded back into the shadows.

Sara was the shining light of the family. She did all she could to please her parents and to spare them aggravation. With all her achievements, however, she never felt satisfied, always aware of a gnawing emptiness inside. She was certain that in some crucial way she was defective.

When she was sixteen, Sara stopped eating. She lived for ten weeks on crackers and water and lost twenty-three pounds. She believed that by starving herself, she could be purged of whatever impurities tainted her. As she became more gaunt and angular, she became obsessed with eradicating the remaining pockets of fat on her body, which she identified with gluttony. When a kidney stone began its painful journey through her body, she embraced the searing pain and gave up her fast.

If Sara was the shining light, her brother, Mark, was the family's thundercloud. At twenty-nine he had already been alcohol-dependent for more than a decade and had accumulated a dozen arrests for driving under the influence of alcohol. From his early teens, he was always in trouble for fighting, truancy, shoplifting, and other run-ins with authority. His hatred for their father was as intense as Sara's devotion. This diversity was partly behind their longstanding estrangement.

As successful as Sara appeared academically, her personal life was a shambles. She had a few girlfriends, but no confidants. She was uneasy around other women and felt that they could not be trusted. Her innermost thoughts and feelings therefore remained private. In her love life, she dove headlong into one infatuation after another. She chose men who were colorful and adventurous. She chose men with charisma who attracted women easily and were unlikely to commit to any one relationship for long. With each one she soon became sexually involved, which led promptly to disillusionment, betrayal, and rage. The intensity of her rage would have been chilling even to the most callous scoundrel.

Sara kept her romantic misadventures secret from her parents. When she was nineteen, in the middle of her sophomore year of college, Sara became pregnant. She panicked at the thought of her father finding out and thought about suicide for weeks before seeking an abortion in a neighboring city. She felt all alone and overcome with guilt and dread as she imagined how disappointed and hurt her father would be if he knew.

4

A House Divided

If a house be divided against itself,
that house cannot stand.

Mark 3:25

"**W**hen it gets too painful to stand, I just go away,"
explained Julie. Julie was a young woman who had
been horribly abused as a child. She had developed the
ability to retreat into a world of fantasy whenever
painful things happened to her body. She would also
"go away" when she felt attacked emotionally. Whenever she felt overwhelmed, she would huddle in a corner, virtually unresponsive for hours or days. Julie
eventually lost her ability to "come back" when it was
safe again. Others use "shutting down" or "numbing
out" to describe the extreme emotional and physical
detachment that they experience under stress.

These are examples of dissociation, a defense
mechanism in which experiences are sorted into compartments that are disconnected from one another. In

this extreme form of discontinuity of experience, memories of feelings or events occurring during one feeling-state may be inaccessible in another. This would be similar to an archeologist examining box after box of fragments of a single great urn, but never recognizing that the contents of one box belong with those of the next.

Less extreme examples of dissociation include daydreaming and "highway hypnosis." People in either state may be fully conscious but oblivious to their surroundings. They may even perform necessary functions, such as driving a car, without paying full attention to what they are doing.

To understand dissociation, think of the brain as a memory recorder with different channels that record and play back information. The channel tuner may be influenced by a number of factors, such as surroundings and mood. Normally, information can be retrieved from more than one channel at a time and integrated. With dissociation, the playback may be confined to a single channel.

For example, a terrifying combat experience may be recorded in memory but stay shut out of awareness after the soldier returns to civilian life. He may later encounter a reminder of his experience, perhaps a threatening situation or a starkly realistic film, such as *Platoon*, that tunes back to the same channel and unlocks the memory. Then he may find himself back in the jungle fighting the enemy, with the real world shut away from consciousness. These flashbacks to traumatic situations are a form of dissociation. Similar flashbacks may occur to terrifying experiences from early childhood.

With multiple personalities, multiple parallel channels are each tuned by a different set of emotional conditions. A personality might be born during a particular kind of traumatic situation that elicits a particular response. The situation may occur once or repeatedly. For example, a frightened child persona might emerge from repeatedly watching parents fight violently, while the child cowers in the corner. A tough punk might emerge from repeatedly being beaten without chance of escape so that the only defense left is to invite the assailant to "lay it on."

Each personality is a two-dimensional caricature adapted to cope with the particular kind of situation for which it was born. Each personality may reemerge and dominate whenever its special strengths are needed or when the current situation resembles in some physical or emotional way the circumstance of that persona's birth. For example, the tough punk might take over in the midst of a sound reprimand from a supervisor at work. While this might help deflect the emotional impact of the reprimand, the resulting behavior might also increase the risk of being fired.

Some of the personalities may be capable of tuning into other channels and becoming aware of their existence. Sometimes the signals get through with interference so that they are perceived as alien voices from within. The discontinuity among personalities is strikingly demonstrated by measurable physical differences, including differences among EEGs (electrical brain wave patterns).

Multiple Personality Disorder is an extreme form of dissociation that is rarely diagnosed. But dissociation is universal among people with BPD.

Annie was a middle-aged attorney who suffered from drastic and sudden mood swings. On one day, she would be filled with energy and enthusiasm, feeling nearly invulnerable. Within hours or days, she would plunge into the depths of despair. Most striking was her total oblivion in each emotional state to the memory of the other.

Annie's mercurial moods were matched by drastic changes in self-esteem and behavior. While euphoric, she would act impulsively without concern for consequences. While despondent, she felt worthless and guilty and would make determined efforts to kill herself.

In order to grow, we must be able to connect our accumulated memories into a consistent picture of the world. Only with such a picture can we make accurate predictions about how our decisions will turn out. If our memories are disconnected from one another, we cannot learn from experience, leaving us at the mercy of our passions. Learning how to reconnect experience is one of the central tasks of therapy.

The Nature of Memory

How literally are childhood memories to be taken? Memory is more like a painting than a photograph. Memories of experiences may be expressionistic, metaphorical, even at times abstract. Moreover, the content of a memory is influenced both by the framework of knowledge through which it is interpreted at the time the experience is recorded, as well as by the intellectual context through which it is expressed at the time of recall.

For example, a child of five may feel intensely jealous of the special bond he perceives between his parents. The nature of this bond may be appreciated only in a nebulous form. When recalled as an adult, however, this jealousy acquires a distinctly and even explicitly sexual context, drawing upon the adult's knowledge of the sexual bond between mates.

Rather than simply a historical narrative of events, memory is constantly undergoing metamorphosis with time and new experience. What results is a layering of impressions that may obscure in crucial ways the essence of the original experience.

The human drive to make sense of our environment further complicates the process. When confronted with loosely related fragments of experience, we tend to fill in the gaps in order to create a more logical picture. Through this kind of revision, the raw material of dreams, which is illogical and bizarre, may be recalled once fully awake in the form of a smoothly coherent story, a story which may vary in detail from telling to telling.

An extreme example of this is seen in a memory disturbance known as Korsakoff's Psychosis. In this condition, often brought on by severe alcoholism combined with nutritional deficiency, the capacity to acquire new knowledge is entirely lost. If we were introduced to an individual so afflicted and left the room for a minute or two, he would have no recollection of the meeting upon our return. When reminded that we have met, however, he would acknowledge the fact and create a fanciful context for how this occurred, which he would perceive as real.

As a medical student, I recall meeting such a patient in the hospital. When I returned after a short absence and prompted him about a previous meeting, he replied without hesitation that we had first met at a Red Sox game at Fenway Park several months earlier and wasn't it a coincidence that we should now find ourselves staying at the same hotel!

While all memory has the potential for subjectivity and inaccuracy (as we have frequently seen portrayed in courtroom dramas), early childhood memories are particularly vulnerable. This vulnerability to distortion increases as we reach back beyond the age at which memory normally develops a sense of continuity over time. This usually occurs between ages seven and ten. Prior to that, we tend to recall only fragments of experience at a time, the earliest fragments generally dating from age two to four.

I recall with great fondness an uncle who died of leukemia when I was five. I can still visualize him vividly in the apartment where he had lived. Are these impressions memories of actual experience or were they created from the many photos I had seen of him, from the many hours I spent in that same apartment until I was nine or ten, and from the many overheard conversations of others in my life who had loved him dearly?

While Freud developed a method of treatment that was based on remembering, he clearly acknowledged that there was no guarantee of the accuracy of the data so produced. Whatever his patient believed, however, was considered crucial to unraveling the genesis of symptoms.

Freud described the complex interplay of mental events that influenced the formation of memories. He understood that memories are in one sense formed at the time that they are first recounted. He noted further that memories, like dreams, may derive partly from substitutions of one idea or object for another and from merging, or condensing, impressions that may have been formed at separate times. Some memories, although vivid, may be more or less fanciful.

In the age of media, personal memories may be further confounded by the bombardment of information and images that we absorb from television and movie screens, personal computers, literature, and music. Bits and pieces of this data may become subliminally incorporated into personal history.

Reconnecting experience may therefore better describe the work of therapy than *recovering memories*. Appreciating the flow of experience from childhood to adulthood is crucial to developing a clear sense of personal identity. As we will see in the next chapter, biological factors may color experience during early childhood development, influence identity, and establish the roots of BPD.

*S*ara's father never found out about her abortion. She seldom
visited home after that, and when she did, she avoided him
as much as possible. She feared that he would see her
shame in her face. When she was twenty-one, early in her senior
year of college, he was killed in a car wreck. When the call came
during the night from her mother, she listened quietly, acknowledged the news, and went back to sleep. When she awoke the next
morning, she remembered the conversation among her dreams
and realized what had happened, but still felt nothing except for
momentary relief that her secret had been preserved.

Sara drifted through the funeral as if in a dream. Even when
she looked at her father in the casket dressed in her favorite suit,
there were no tears. Some of her relatives were appalled by her
apparent lack of feelings, while others were concerned, anticipating a storm of feelings when the reality of her loss finally hit her.
Mark showed up late, half drunk, and Sara barely noticed him
there. Oddly, he seemed more troubled by their father's tragic
death than she.

The emotional storm never came. Soon after her father's
death, Sara met Jonathan, and they were married within
months. Jonathan was thirty-two when they met. He was different from most of the other men with whom she had become
involved. He was only slightly taller than she. His pale com-
plexion, blond hair, and grey eyes blended to form a pleasant
face, but he lacked the ruggedness that had attracted her to
most of her former lovers. He was serious and responsible and
appeared dedicated to his work. He worked as a paramedic and
became most animated when telling tales of harrowing rescues,
which Sara enjoyed hearing. His work was the one thing about
him that she found exciting.

Jonathan had been married once before. After three years of
marriage, his wife had begun to drink heavily and eventually
left him for another man. Jonathan had been deeply hurt. He
had not dated for the two years following the divorce, and then
he was introduced to Sara. He fell deeply in love with her at

once. She was charmed by his devotion to her and felt comfortable and secure with him, but she did not love him with the passion of earlier romances.

Sara and Jonathan lived peacefully together during their early years of marriage. Sara became as driven in her career as Jonathan was in his. She often brought work home and worked far into the night while Jonathan slept. When they occasionally spent an evening or a Sunday afternoon together, they shared victories and defeats from their working lives and encouraged each other. They seldom spoke of other things.

One night Jonathan came home particularly shaken. His ambulance had been called to the scene of a shooting. When they arrived, they had found a little boy of five or six bleeding from a chest wound and barely breathing. They had gotten him to the hospital, but he doubted the child would survive. The child's distraught mother had explained how the accident had occurred. But Jonathan had an uneasy feeling about the man who was with her. This man had glared at the woman as she spoke, and she had glanced nervously at him after every sentence as if looking for his approval.

Sara felt sick to her stomach when Jonathan concluded his story. She ran to the bathroom and retched. She would not let Jonathan near her to comfort her and rocked through the night, dozing toward morning.

The next day Sara left for work as usual but never showed up. When she pulled into their driveway at dusk, more than two hundred miles had registered on the speedometer. But Sara had no idea at all where she had been.

5

Suffer the Little Children

Origins of Borderline Personality Disorder

Love and pain can be one and the same
In the eyes of a wounded child.

"HELL IS FOR CHILDREN"
PAT BENETAR, NEIL GERALDO, ROGER CAPPS

Until recently, the debate about the origins of BPD was primarily between those who believed it was a biological disorder and those who believed it represented a failure of early childhood development. This would be like archeologists debating about whether the characteristics of an ancient pot derived more from the qualities of the clay from which it was formed or from the technique of the potter.

The biologists supported their beliefs with findings that relatives of patients with BPD had a greater than average incidence of certain mood disorders. They also found physiologic similarities between patients with BPD and those with biological depression. For example, both groups had a shortened time from the onset of sleep to the onset of the rapid eye movement (REM), or dreaming stage, of sleep.

Psychoanalytic theory attributes emotional problems in adulthood to problems in completing developmental steps as a child. After describing the problems that people with BPD have with relationships, psychoanalysts identified the developmental stages during which these issues are normally addressed. This is akin to examining the flaws in a pot and deciding whether they occurred during the molding, the glazing, or the firing.

If you are borderline, you lack an enduring trust in the goodness of your love objects and yourself; you have little tolerance for flaws in yourself or others, and you are unable to comfort yourself while alone.

The establishment of fundamental trust in a caretaker, even when absent, inconsistent, or frustrating, is usually accomplished toward the end of the second year of life. During this stage, the child begins to recognize and accept that while Mama sometimes says "no," she still can be relied on when it counts. It is also during this stage that the child finds ways to soothe herself when the caretaker is not around, often with the help of a treasured comfort-object, such as a blanket or teddy bear. It is, in fact, common among people with BPD not to recall ever having a special comfort-object.

During the same stage, the child develops an awareness of an identity separate from the caretaker, and she begins to develop confidence in her ability to explore the world on her own. If she is guided gently and allowed to take some risks while being protected from serious danger, her feelings of competence and security will flourish. If she is criticized and punished for venturing out, she is likely to feel inadequate and insecure and to remain dependent on others.

Such apparent failures of development were once attributed solely to faulty parenting at the relevant developmental stage. Today we understand that biology and experience, "nature" and "nurture," together may influence development. Innate differences in temperament can significantly influence the parent-child relationship. For example, inborn differences in frustration-tolerance would affect a child's interpretation of how well her needs were being met, and would affect the parent's emotional response to the child.

More recently, the role of major traumatic events in childhood and adolescence has been recognized as contributing to BPD. Four out of five patients with BPD have a clear history of strikingly traumatic experiences. An overwhelming majority of these have been physically abused and a similar number have been sexually abused. Many have witnessed severe violence among others in their household. Most commonly, they have been traumatized repeatedly and in more than one way. Physical and sexual abuse frequently occur together.

Some investigators believe that BPD can be explained as the natural outcome of such events. Defenses such as splitting and dissociation could certainly arise in the face of overwhelming danger, particularly at the hands of a caretaker or other valued person. Instead of a failure to develop trust, a loss of trust once held would be a natural consequence of betrayal.

Such theories emphasize destructive forces in much the same way an archeologist might compare the effects of erosion on differently made vessels and conclude that the effects of the environment were more important determinants of the final appearance than the manner of creation.

Which theory makes the most sense? BPD is a complex disorder that probably derives from a complex interplay of biological and experiential factors. It may actually represent a common behavioral expression of a variety of underlying problems. For example, for some people with BPD, the genetic link with depression may be more prominent and the experience of physical or sexual abuse less frequent.

We must also acknowledge that the factors discussed are not independent. While some people with BPD have been abused by outsiders, many have suffered at the hands of close family members who were also influential during critical early development. Furthermore, there may be biological factors in common that predispose a child to becoming borderline that may also lead other family members to be moody, inconsistent, or abusive. Finally, since abuse tends to be passed from generation to generation, common experiences may account for an unusually high incidence of both BPD and mood instability in some families.

Christine was thirty-three when she was first admitted to a psychiatric hospital following an overdose of drugs. This had occurred in the aftermath of her divorce from an abusive husband. In addition to depressed mood, she also complained of severe and persistent headaches for which she was taking considerable amounts of narcotic pain-relieving medications. She reported a history of accident-proneness with a remarkable number of broken bones and other less severe injuries. Her mood fluctuated wildly. At times she was docile and friendly. At other times she voiced vitriolic rage. She sometimes "lost" time, with periods of hours for which she was unable to account. Some of her injuries appeared mysteriously during such times.

When first seen, Christine could recall little of her early childhood. She did not recall being abused in any way. She did remember a single episode of attempted molestation by a neighbor at age sixteen after she had been baby-sitting for his child, but she expressed little concern about this incident. Christine reported no known history of emotional problems in her family, but she knew little about her mother's family, which lived in a distant part of the country.

After almost two years of treatment, Christine attended a reunion of her mother's family. At her next session, she excitedly told me that all five of the female first cousins she met were just like her. In fact, she boasted, she was the healthiest one of them all. They all suffered from both mood swings and headaches. Three had attempted suicide. Two others were accident-prone and one cut herself repeatedly on the thighs with a razor blade. Headaches and moodiness had begun to show up in several of their teenage daughters. Of her male cousins, none admitted to headaches or emotional instability, but she observed several become staggeringly drunk at the gathering.

Christine's story illustrates the apparent inheritance of BPD in some families. In her family, the women typically developed symptoms of BPD while the men showed a strong tendency toward alcoholism. These may both be expressions of a single underlying disturbance of the nervous system. Her story also illustrates the danger of assuming that childhood trauma is always behind BPD.

If we examine an ancient artifact, we can appreciate that all the factors we have discussed have contributed to its present condition. Both the quality of the clay and the skill of the potter influenced the original form and character of the piece. These factors also helped determine its resistance to the ravages of time and the elements. While each factor may be considered separately in order to comprehend its influence, we must be aware of how they have interacted if we are to appreciate fully the complexity of the object we behold.

A Word About Gender

Throughout this book, I have generally used the feminine pronoun when talking about people with BPD. This is in keeping with the preponderance of women with this diagnosis. While this may reflect some observer bias, it is most likely a valid finding.

Why would BPD be a particularly feminine problem? Sex role differences may be one factor. Culturally and biologically, men have a greater tendency than women to act out aggression directly toward others. Women more often refrain from outwardly directed aggression, either turning it against themselves or expressing it indirectly. This leads to the self-destructive behaviors that most typically characterize BPD.

Men have traditionally worked out aggression in competitive contact sports, both as participants and spectators, by hunting, in military action, and by competition in business. Less acceptable outlets include barroom brawls, gang wars, armed robbery, domestic violence, and other illegal activities.

Men more often take physical risks, engage in reckless activities, or provoke retaliation by others. These often self-defeating behaviors may be equivalent emotionally to the deliberate self-injury that is the hallmark of BPD. Accident-proneness may be a covert form of self-injury in both men and women.

Recklessness is one of the characteristics of Antisocial Personality Disorder. While there are a number of outward differences between antisocial and borderline personalities, both experience intense emotional distress and have unstable, short-lived relationships. The preponderance of men among people with antisocial personalities parallels the excess of women among people with BPD.

Excessive drinking may be another camouflage for borderline dynamics in men. Alcohol is mood altering and is often used impulsively in response to rejection, anger, and loneliness. Drinking can be self-injurious and often leads to more overtly reckless behavior. Drinking also serves to maintain emotional distance in relationships.

To the extent that sexual molestation and rape play a causative role in BPD, the preponderance of women so affected would make sense. Women are more often victims of sexual crimes. This difference is perhaps exaggerated by a relatively greater underreporting of these crimes by men.

Finally, the last several decades have brought a growing blur of gender role boundaries. This may contribute to the fragmented, mercurial identity that is part of being borderline. This blurring of gender roles has clearly affected both men and women, but has perhaps required a greater degree of change and adjustment in women's lifestyles and identities. The overwhelming array of choices and competing demands for time and attention that women must face today expose them to confusion and doubt about who they are and what is meaningful to them.

A Word to Male Readers

Despite the emphasis on women in this book, many men suffer from BPD and related disorders. Please read on and change the pronouns mentally if it helps you to identify more closely.

As you read, you may also find other substitutions helpful. For example, combat trauma may have emotional effects closely resembling those of childhood abuse. Dissociation is a common response to both kinds of trauma. Post-traumatic Stress Disorder, a frequently diagnosed condition among combat veterans, bears a striking resemblance in some of its aspects to BPD.

If you have difficulty controlling aggressive impulses, read the chapters on impulse and self-mutilation with this in mind. What you learn about the mood-altering effects of these behaviors may be helpful in learning to tame your rage.

Whether or not you are borderline, by reading this book you hopefully will acquire valuable knowledge about the origins of your emotional pain that will help you to control it.

We have learned how traumatic experiences can contribute to the development of borderline symptoms in both men and women. Exposure to overwhelming danger from which there is no possibility of escape can lead to overwhelming fear and rage and can activate emotional defenses that help modify the intensity of these feelings. In the next chapter, we will look more closely at the specific role of sexual victimization in the development of symptoms.

*A*fter our first meeting, Sara was admitted to an alcohol and drug treatment program. We began to schedule therapy sessions before she was discharged and continued to meet weekly in my office. She was initially guarded and mistrustful, but soon became more comfortable. She talked more and more freely about her life and feelings. It seemed that the most intriguing bits of her story were often left for the end of the session, enticing me to spill over just a little into the next patient's time. When I would interrupt her at such times, she would leave the office begrudgingly. Invariably the opportunity would appear lost as the next session veered off in a different direction. On the few occasions that I yielded to the temptation to let her go on, she would soon digress and lead me down a blind path.

About eight months into treatment, Sara first shared a recurring nightmare. In the dream, she is walking in a pine forest. It is a beautiful fall day. She is enjoying the solitude. Dusk falls more quickly than she expected and she discovers she is lost. There is no longer a path and the forest looks the same in all directions. She begins to run. Finally she can make out a figure in the distance, but all of a sudden she hears the "whack! whack!" of a woodsman's ax and a tree falls in her path. More trees begin to fall all around her. She is hopelessly hemmed in. The figure in the distance can no longer be seen. She is alone and terrified.

As time passed, Sara's nightmare recurred over and over. Each time we revisited it, it had changed in some detail. One day I asked her to imagine herself back in the dream, but to experience it from the viewpoint of the distant figure. She managed this shift in perspective easily. She was searching, she said, for a missing child. She was very apprehensive because the child was very small. Sara expressed surprise because she had not previously been aware that in the dream she was a child. As she continued to search for the child, trees began to fall around her. She was frightened that the child would be hurt, but then became too occupied with avoiding the falling trees to give the child more thought.

Sara's heart was racing. She talked more and more excitedly as the account went on. She began to feel sick and remembered the wounded child in Jonathan's story. Then, for the first time, she wept.

6 | *Crimes Without Punishment / Punishment Without Crimes*

Look at the ceiling
The shadows are bears
In hurricanes where do birds hide
When Daddy's hands rub me all over, I wonder
Where butterflies learn how to fly?

"Look at the Ceiling"
from *Uniforms*
Peter Alsop

If you are borderline, you were likely victimized at some time. Physical and sexual abuse are easiest to identify. Children also are abused when they are made to witness violence, when they are exposed to danger or terror, or when they are cruelly imprisoned, for example, by being bound or confined in a small place.

These experiences are often hidden away in a remote corner of memory until something triggers a connection, a reminder of old horrors. Therapy itself may stir up these memories and bring them into the light. At some point in therapy, you are likely to explore this corner of your personal history. This task should be undertaken with caution and respect.

Why try to remember at all? Because these powerful experiences are linked to present-day distortions of reality. They may cripple your capacity to trust others, to enjoy intimacy, to value yourself, and to permit your creativity to blossom. They may hamper your growth emotionally, intellectually, spiritually, and even physically.

Remembering can be enlightening and rewarding, but it also can be painful and destructive. How the remembering occurs is crucial to its outcome. Your relationship with your therapist, your guide in this quest, is also critically important. Sufficient trust should be built between the two of you before beginning the journey.

The feelings you have for your therapist should be closely monitored throughout the process. If you experience your therapist as critical, punishing, or intrusive, these feelings must be discussed until their origins become clear. Such feelings may present a key to understanding other distortions of present-day reality.

Remembering by itself is not sufficient for healing to occur. However, remembering painful experiences in the secure presence of a trusted caretaker is crucial to the healing process. Exploration should be gentle and gradual. A headlong rush into the past may result in an emotional reenactment of the original abuse, with the therapist as onlooker. Both you and your therapist must be vigilant in preventing this. Pacing therapy is the joint responsibility of you and your therapist.

We have already seen how memories can be influenced by the context in which they are evoked. Therapy can itself be a powerful force in shaping memory. It is crucial that neither you nor your therapist assume too much about what you may find. Pursuing a simple answer to your suffering can be very appealing, but can also be dangerously misleading. Beware of any therapist who insists that one thing or another must have happened to you based solely on your presenting symptoms.

If you think you have been abused and plan to explore your history, formal psychotherapy is strongly advised. While books are available to help guide your exploration, they can evoke powerful emotions and sometimes mislead. Books are best used with the help of a personal guide. Support groups for exploring abuse also can be helpful, but these also present hazards if they are used alone. Your pace may not be the same as that of others in the group, and you may experience floods of emotion for which you are unprepared.

The object of exploration is to put painful memories to rest and allow you to live more peacefully in the present. This purpose must be kept clearly in mind. Therapy can be misused to justify clinging to symptoms, to exact revenge on others, or to punish yourself by reenacting the original trauma over and over again.

Guilt

Guilt is the most bewildering emotion facing the survivor of abuse. Terror, rage, and despair are powerful, but they are fitting and understandable. A victim's guilt is equally compelling and more difficult to resolve because of its apparently illogical origins.

It is natural for others to reassure victims of their blamelessness when they express guilt. Reassurances of this sort are seldom reassuring. When offered by therapists, they often lead to more emphatic declarations of guilt. Why? Because they deny the authenticity of your feelings. Having your feelings acknowledged and respected is part of healing.

If you are allowed to experience your guilty feelings, you may learn more about their origins, permitting you finally to put them to rest. In order to understand these origins as an adult, you will need to keep in mind that these events were experienced by a child.

To a child, crime and punishment are inseparable. Horrible suffering must be deserved. Only bad children get punished. These deeply held beliefs may be reinforced by the perpetrator of abuse by telling the child she is naughty and deserves to be punished. In order to enforce secrecy, the abuser may even tell the child that the things that they did together are naughty and must be kept secret. Such brainwashing is one of the most insidious aspects of child abuse.

Sometimes the circumstances of victimization may emphasize the connection with punishment. For example, a child being punished for a minor offense was left behind from a family outing. On this occasion, she was sexually molested by the babysitter and came to believe she deserved it.

Repeated victimization by more than one abuser particularly underscores feelings of guilt and defectiveness. Each episode feels like a punishment for the ones before and a confirmation of dirtiness. Why else would one child be singled out over and over?

Child molesters are human predators, and predators go after wounded prey. Like the bass that is particularly attracted to the crippled minnow or the shark attracted to blood, molesters are sensitive to the signs of vulnerability that result from previous victimization.

Others may reinforce the child's feelings of shame by laying blame or simply by failing to help. For example, attempts to tell a parent about abuse may be met with denial by the parent or accusations that the child is lying, has a dirty mind, or is responsible for whatever happened to her. Some parents may know about or even witness episodes of abuse. By failing to intervene, they tacitly participate, leaving the child feeling abandoned, worthless, and bewildered.

Sexual abuse may create mixed feelings that arouse guilt. Genital stimulation may produce sexual arousal and pleasurable sensations even in the presence of fear. These physiologic responses are involuntary reflexes that have developed in the course of evolution. To the child, however, they may be perceived as forbidden pleasure.

The child may perceive other forbidden gains accompanying sexual abuse. If the abuser is a parent or caretaker, the abuse may be the most attention the child has had from that person.

Coercion comes in many guises. To a child, withholding attention can be a powerful form of coercion. Sexual molestation may be accompanied by physical expressions of affection that are sometimes the only affection the child receives. The abuser also may bribe the child with candy or other concrete rewards to participate in sexual acts.

When a child experiences pleasure or perceives gain from participating in forbidden acts, guilt is sure to follow. Guilt may follow despite the overwhelming advantage an adult has over a child. That advantage blurs any distinction between persuasion and coercion.

When an abuser is a parent or family member, he or she cannot simply become the enemy. A child is in no position to discard a parent who has betrayed her. Deep longing for closeness and affection may continue even in the face of rage. Rage must be denied when it threatens a relationship that the child is desperate to preserve. One way to do this is to reassign blame: "Someone here is responsible for these bad things that have happened. It can't be Daddy, so it must be me." The rage is converted into guilt in order to avoid destroying something that is valued.

You may recognize here the defense of splitting. In this case, the child has split away the badness of a loved person and accepted it for herself. Guilt, in this case, protects the child from experiencing the more painful feelings of loneliness and abandonment. Guilt may also defend the child against overwhelming feelings of powerlessness. It accompanies an illusion of power and choice that may also be reflected in heroic fantasies of escape or triumph.

Gwendolyn was a twenty-nine-year-old woman who had been repeatedly molested by her attorney father between the ages of eight and eleven. She entered treatment when she was hospitalized for a suicide attempt prompted by a failing marriage. Early in treatment, Gwen began to remember how she was molested. Even as she expressed rage and fear toward her father, she longed for him to visit her in the hospital and was bitterly disappointed at his lack of interest in her. When she was well on the road to recovery and seeking to further her education, she became a legal assistant and later went on to law school.

Gwen had been filled with self-loathing and guilt. It was remarkably ironic that her growing self-esteem should be rooted in her identification with the profession of the father who had betrayed her.

With an incisive wit, Gwendolyn once told me, "You are what you can't beat." She was commenting on the pervasive effects of victimhood on identity. I think she was also saying how hard it is for a victim to keep her own identity distinct from that of her abuser and to avoid taking on the guilt for his transgressions.

Sexual abuse has been emphasized in this chapter more than other forms of abuse not only because of the frequency with which it appears among my patients, but also because of the complexity of feelings that arise around it. Examining the emotional responses to molestation provides a framework for understanding the effects of other kinds of trauma.

During the last decade, there has been a dramatic increase in public awareness of the scope of child abuse in our society. This has led to expanded advocacy of children and hopefully prevention of much abuse. It has also resulted in public accusations of parents by adult children and quests for revenge that have often had disastrous results, including splintered families.

More recently, a vocal group of parents of alleged victims of incest have vigorously denied their children's accusations and proposed a False Memory Syndrome as the origin of such memories. They have accused therapists of planting the concept of abuse in patients' minds deliberately. In at least one such case, a parent sued his daughter's therapists for malpractice and won a substantial award. This backlash has called into question the validity of all therapy concerned with childhood memories. Whether or not repression and later recovery of memories of traumatic events can occur has even been questioned.

There is no doubt that painful events can be blocked from conscious awareness. Dissociation, as we have already seen, is one way this can occur, even with repeated trauma. While memory is admittedly subjective and imperfect, recall can be validated in many cases. I have treated patients whose memories of abuse, which have sometimes emerged after decades of oblivion, have been corroborated by other victims within the same family, including younger victims whose experiences were contemporary or had never been forgotten. With other patients, the internal consistency and emotional tone of their developing histories has been convincing.

I have also treated patients who, under the influence of self-help groups, the media, or prior therapists, have jumped to early conclusions about victimization that have been unconvincing. In these cases, it has been my delicate task to help my patients question their conclusions while still validating their feelings.

Hypnosis has been implicated by the "false memory" movement as a dangerous technique that generates misleading data. What can be misleading is the assumption that data recalled under hypnosis has particular validity. I believe that memories evoked under hypnosis are neither more nor less valid than those evoked in the waking state. What is crucial in both instances is that the inquiry be unbiased. Questions that lead or insinuate have no more place during hypnosis than during a waking therapeutic interview. Both patient and therapist must understand the limitations of memory in either state and be willing to consider alternative interpretations of the data.

Finally, it is not only victims who may develop amnesia for an event. In some cases, perpetrators may not remember what they have done. Abusive acts may be committed in dissociative states that have been facilitated by their own history as victims. Alcohol is frequently a factor that leads to abusive behavior. When sufficiently intoxicated, events may be blacked out by amnesia once the effects of alcohol have worn off. This chemically induced state is akin to dissociation. Whether through drinking or dissociation, some perpetrators may remain totally unaware of their own deeds.

Like the archeologist who discovers an isolated artifact from a lost civilization, we must be cautious about the conclusions we draw from fragments of memory. Patience is required in both endeavors so that a context can be gradually developed that will clarify the meaning of the clue.

While the groundwork for BPD may be laid early in childhood, symptoms may not appear until well into adulthood. We will see next how new experiences may arouse feelings attached to earlier traumatic experiences and trigger the beginning of symptoms.

*S*ara was late to her next session. She had expected me to be angry. In fact, she imagined that I would not see her at all that day. She felt embarrassed about having cried the previous session. She did not feel that treatment was getting anywhere and was thinking about stopping. She was afraid she was wasting my time and Jonathan's money. She was certain that she was the most hopeless patient I had ever treated. I would be entirely justified if I discharged her.

When I asked her to clarify who was discharging whom, Sara fell silent. Her emotions changed from guilt to anger. She asked why I was putting her through so much pain if I didn't know how to fix her. Why couldn't she just go back to using the Valium and wine that I had taken away from her? Then she could at least get momentary relief. She had felt frightened by the dream images, and she had imagined that I would rescue her and put a stop to the nightmares. She had felt so alone and helpless at the end of the previous session that she had wanted to stay with me a while longer. When I did not invite her to do so, she had felt entirely abandoned.

We were to learn that Sara's nightmare contained many layers of meaning. At this point in her treatment, the most important meaning was the metaphor it contained for the treatment itself. Sara had begun her journey in therapy with hope. As she wandered into the forest, she initially felt cared for and protected, but soon became overwhelmed by the seeming endlessness of the undertaking. She began to fear that I would not be there long enough to help her see it through. And there was no turning back.

As Sara discussed her terror of being left to deal on her own with all her painful feelings, her anger subsided. She had felt reassured to find me waiting for her when she was late. We reaffirmed our agreement to work together until she felt strong enough to manage her life without me. Our next session would confirm that she now felt safe enough to allow the memories to surface.

7

The Beginning of Symptoms

*Ophelia: There's rosemary, that's for remembrance—
pray you love, remember—and there is pansies,
that's for thoughts.*

*Laertes: A document in madness, thoughts and
remembrance fitted.*

HAMLET, ACT IV, SCENE V.

A tell is a hill that contains the ruins of many civilizations, each built upon the ruins of the one before. The appearance of a tell rising starkly against a flat landscape is a clue to the existence of the secrets within. So symptoms appear as markers that signify critical events that have occurred in our personal histories. Often the symptoms themselves will contain important clues to the nature and timing of these events.

While personality disorders usually imply lifelong behavior patterns, many people first develop borderline symptoms in adulthood. For others, an isolated crisis in adolescence may be followed by years of relatively stable functioning before symptoms recur.

If you are borderline, there are many ways that you can tame the chaos that rages within. External structure can compensate for your lack of consistent internal values. Many people with BPD successfully embed

49

themselves within systems that have clear-cut rules and routines. Some enlist in the military. Others become members of religious cults or sects whose rigid rules and values greatly simplify day-to-day decision making.

Selecting a dominant partner is another way to simplify choices and create a sense of continuity, although at the expense of being stifled or even abused. This strategy may work well until something disrupts the relationship, leaving you suddenly directionless.

Selecting a demanding vocation can also lend stability and consistency. Many people with latent BPD are workaholics. By immersing themselves in highly demanding jobs, they accept powerful one-dimensional identities that can be sustained as long as they can keep up performance. When emotional defenses are working effectively, not only can painful emotions be kept in check, but also painful memories. Painful childhood experiences, such as physical or sexual abuse, frequently escape awareness for years, sometimes reemerging at times of emotional crisis. When such memories surface, they often carry an impact similar to the original experience.

It is possible, therefore, to establish a delicate balance in which life appears normal, untouched by catastrophic childhood experiences or genetic vulnerability. When the balance is finally disturbed, it is often like a volcanic eruption, scalding everything in its path. The tremendous energy that once worked to contain painful emotions now fuels these emotions and the impulses that accompany them.

Many kinds of events can upset the balance and release the destructive energy. Consider the effects of a physical injury. An injury may interfere with the ability to work. This interrupts routine, disrupts roles that may have become crucial to identity, and creates financial hardship. The injury itself may cause physical pain or deformity. For BPD victims, an injury is a violation of body boundaries that may reawaken feelings attached to earlier experiences of physical or sexual abuse.

Treatment of an injury requires investing trust in an authority figure. This may be particularly difficult in the face of earlier betrayals. The accompanying feelings of helplessness may also reopen old wounds. Treatment often also includes use of mind-altering medications, such as narcotic pain medications, that can affect mood and impair self-control.

Finally, if legal action is involved, the victim of the injury may be accused of lying about its severity or of contributing to its occurrence. This may also recreate aspects of earlier experiences as a victim.

If there has been abuse in childhood, any reminder of that abuse could trigger a crisis. New experiences that bear some real or symbolic resemblance to the original trauma can revive old feelings. For example, adult sexual intimacy can revive fears that originated with childhood sexual abuse. Anniversaries of important events can also trigger connections.

Belinda was a middle-aged woman who became depressed and self-destructive each year at Easter. She had been molested first by her grandfather at age six during a family visit after Easter church services.

Barbara attempted suicide for the first time at age thirty-three, shortly after her oldest daughter's eighth birthday. She had had her first incestuous encounter with her father at age eight.

Maryellen was overcome by panic while on a boat fishing with her fiance. Her terror was explained later by flashbacks of a similar fishing trip at age seven when she had watched a cousin drown.

Whether it is an anniversary or symbolic event, a painful current experience, a loss, a stressful change, or an interruption of routine that first unleashes powerful old feelings and memories, these feelings are not likely to go back into hiding.

If you were an adult when symptoms first broke through, you have probably developed relationships and roles that fit you well. These roles came to define you. Now they no longer fit at all. The once comforting routine of your job may now feel empty and oppressive. The lover or marital partner that once provided you guidance and security now feels domineering and smothering.

Sex has perhaps become an ordeal, particularly if memories of sexual abuse have recently come to light. What had once been a normal part of your love relationships may now feel like a recurring assault upon your body's boundaries, further estranging you from your partner.

With the beginning of symptoms, therefore, comes an avalanche of losses, which may leave you feeling empty, helpless, and alone. While you may be able to save important relationships, these have been irrevocably changed and are only remnants of the past. You must grieve for these losses and changes before you can grow into new and more fulfilling roles in love, work, and faith.

*T*he night before the following session, Sara called in a frenzy. She had been putting her children to bed when she suddenly saw a vivid image of her own bedroom from when she was around their age. This rare glimpse of her early childhood was accompanied by a terror that left her bewildered. She described the room to me excitedly. There was a window seat in a dormer window that identified it as an upstairs bedroom. A wooden toy chest with a teddy bear painted on the lid sat in a corner of the room. A whole family of teddy bears slept with her in her bed.

Sara's family had moved from this house when she was eight. She had often struggled to visualize it, but could extract no trace of it from her memory. Now the picture had suddenly come alive and become unmistakably familiar. The terror was also hauntingly familiar. As she spoke, the fear began to subside and she accepted my reassurance that we would talk more the following morning.

When Sara sat in my office the next day, the memories continued to surface. As she described in great detail not only her room, but the whole house in which she had grown up, she was once again overcome with panic. But this time her fear was accompanied by a terrifying memory.

One night when she was four years old, Sara was awakened from sleep as her daddy's arm swept her by the waist from her bed and carried her downstairs. Her head barely missed hitting the bannister as her daddy ran down the stairs. While his powerful arm still encircled her, she saw something metallic flash in the air and felt something very hard press against her temple.

Sara's mommy was in the living room. She was crying and looked very frightened. Her daddy was screaming something at her mommy, who seemed to be begging. Her daddy's breath smelled like medicine and made her sick. Sara closed her eyes, froze, and tried to shut out the terror. He finally let go of her and *the hard object was gone. She opened her eyes just in time to see him whack her mommy sharply across the face with the back of his hand, then again with his palm.*

This scene repeated many times. Sara began lying awake deep into the night, praying that he wouldn't come. She became familiar with the sickening alcohol smell that permeated these terrifying scenes. She dreaded the sensation of the gun barrel against her head while he demanded that her mommy admit that she was cheating on him. She watched the terror in her mommy's eyes as he threatened to pull the trigger.

When the gun finally drew away from her head, there was always a moment of relief before she heard the "whack! whack!" that left her mommy sobbing on the floor.

After a while Sara learned how to shut the scene out and escape mentally from the fear. She would focus on a favorite tune and play it over and over in her head. Her daddy's angry voice and her mommy's sobs would become distant, fading to an indistinct murmur. Eventually she learned to "go away" at will.

8

In the Looking Glass

Who Looks Back?

*". . . was I the same when I got up this morning? I
almost think I can remember feeling a little different.
But if I'm not the same, the next question is, Who in
the world am I? Ah, that's the great puzzle!"*

*"I'm sure I'm not Ada," she said, "for her hair goes in
such long ringlets, and mine doesn't go in ringlets at
all; and I'm sure I can't be Mabel, for I know all sorts
of things and she, oh! she knows such a very little!
Besides, she's she, and I'm I, and—oh dear, how puz-
zling it all is!"*

ALICE'S ADVENTURES IN WONDERLAND
LEWIS CARROLL

If you are borderline, you are in a constant search for
clues about who you are. You struggle with a vague
feeling of insubstantiality and may feel, at times, that
you could suddenly vanish. You may cling to relationships in a desperate attempt to maintain a frame of reference for your own identity.

Whether you are borderline or not, your experience of the world is unique. Every perception is fil-
tered through the totality of all your previous
experiences so that it has special meaning for you.

When you look at a rose, you see the same flower that others
see, but you may respond more through your sense of smell,
while someone else is struck by the rose's velvety texture. You
may flash back to the trellis in the backyard of your childhood
home, while someone else is reminded of their favorite rock
band. The complexity and individuality of response to even a single image is astonishing.

Knowing yourself is understanding the boundaries of your
experience. This means appreciating how you are distinct from
others as well as how you experience things similarly.

Imagine being alone in a country in which a language is spoken that you do not understand at all. Conversation is going on
all around you. People are laughing and gesturing, thoroughly
engaged with one another. You probably feel left out and perhaps
envious of the easy warmth with which others are conversing.
You may also feel apprehensive, wondering how you will find
your way around this strange place without language to guide
you. You may feel excited to be embarking on a new adventure.

Your own nationality and language have suddenly become
very apparent to you. As you look around, you also become
aware of how your own facial features and mannerisms and those
of your friends and family differ from those of these strange for-
eigners. Of course, here you are the foreigner, a crucial part of
your identity for the moment. You may also imagine what it
would feel like to be back home surrounded by friends and deep
in conversation. The emotional response that this evokes is also
part of your identity and may germinate feelings of kinship with
the strangers around you.

If you stay long enough, you will begin to learn the native language and customs. With time, you may even begin to think in
your new language, a major transformation of experience.

Upon your next arrival at the same destination, your experience will be drastically different. In place of strangeness will be
familiarity of language, place, and perhaps even faces. The feelings evoked by this familiar place will be strongly influenced by

your experiences during the previous trip, experiences that have now woven themselves into your identity.

Identity is fluid, ever changing. Aspects of identity, like ethnicity or nationality, sit largely in the background until circumstances focus attention upon them. There is a constant flow of features into the limelight and back into the wings.

Identity is also constantly changing with new experiences. Aging brings some of the most profound changes in the way we view ourselves. Our bodies transform drastically as we move from infancy to old age. And yet, we miraculously retain a sense of continuity and oneness.

What is it that enables friends to recognize us at a distance when they have not seen us in twenty-five years and perhaps twice as many pounds? And how is it that warm (or angry) feelings can stir suddenly upon seeing a familiar face from the past? Something enduring about how we think, feel, move, and speak transcends all the adjustments that are made to identity over the years.

Identity is a blend of enduring features and the growing collage of experience that we accumulate through life. The more comfortable we feel with the enduring aspects of our identities, the more accepting we are likely to be of the inevitable changes that come with time.

You already know a lot about yourself. Consider only a few of the possible dimensions you can measure. Where were you born? Where did you grow up? Where are your parents from? your grandparents? In what religion were you raised? What are your current beliefs? What are your favorite foods, colors, kinds of music? How tall are you? Where are you in the birth order of your family? How quick are you to anger? Are you embarrassed when you cry? How were you educated? Do you learn better with your ears, eyes, or hands?

By asking yourself questions about features ranging from physical characteristics to moral values, you can develop an intricately detailed self-portrait, which is the beginning of identity. As you examine the portrait, you will have feelings about each of the qualities you identify. These feelings form another layer of identity.

Fundamental to a sense of wholeness, however, are your feelings of being loved and valued by others and your perception of how well your personal boundaries have been respected.

Boundaries include the boundaries of your body, as well as your thoughts and feelings. Physical and sexual abuse are clear violations of body boundaries. A parent telling a child when she is hungry or cold rather than allowing the child to identify those feelings is a more subtle violation of emotional boundaries.

Clear boundaries are based upon your accurate communication and the willingness of another person to hear and validate what you have communicated. This means that when you express an emotion, the other person acknowledges that is how you feel and respects your right to feel that way.

If you are borderline, some of your boundaries may have been severely violated. You have been accustomed to your words being ineffective and have responded to the powerlessness of words by translating feelings into action. If your physical boundaries have been violated, you may desperately try to redefine the limits of your body by cutting your skin. You may meticulously control what you allow to enter your body, including its nourishment. You may even experiment with changing the boundaries, like Alice, by altering your body's size.

If you are borderline, you may experience identifications with others as an intrusion. If you have been abused by a family member, you may feel appalled at your genetic endowment and despise any aspect of your abuser that you detect in yourself. You may even try to destroy that part of you through suicide or self-mutilation.

Boundaries are also violated when others partake too fully of our emotions and lay claim to them as their own. One episode of the original Star Trek series featured alien creatures called Empaths. These creatures picked up the emotions of others intuitively, and exquisitely, painfully, and even fatally experienced them. If you are borderline, you may sometimes perceive others as Empaths and may at times feel like one yourself: unable to observe feelings without experiencing them.

When relationships have adequate boundaries, feelings can be communicated without fear either of injuring others or of reprisal. Your feelings remain yours, even if they are similar to someone else's. You may imagine yourself in another's shoes, but you do not walk in those shoes, nor do you expect others to walk in yours.

Developing sound boundaries depends both on how you choose relationships and how you communicate within them. If you are borderline, you probably grew up in a family in which boundaries were fuzzy and poorly respected. You probably are still attracted to people whose boundaries are ill-defined and who may become intrusive or abusive. As you develop your boundaries and learn to protect them through accurate and timely communication of feelings and expectations, you will learn to discern at an early stage whether someone is unwilling or incapable of respecting your limits, and you will move on to more emotionally nourishing relationships.

Jenny was a thirty-four-year-old mother of three. She began working part-time for an accounting firm when her youngest child began nursery school. She was originally hired for half-time, but several coworkers regularly asked her to do extra work that kept her in the office longer and longer. By the end of a year, she was working forty hours per week and the workload was still growing. Jenny approached her supervisor to let her know how overwhelmed she felt. The supervisor reassured her that she was doing an excellent job. She had no doubt that Jenny would handle even greater responsibility as time went on.

As the work load grew, Jenny became more and more irritable. Her family doctor prescribed tranquilizers and reassured her that she would get over her moodiness. She took increasing amounts of the tranquilizers. She soon began scratching her thighs in neatly spaced lines with a razor blade during her lunch break. One Saturday morning, her boss called her to work on a special project. Jenny agreed and, during a coffee break, cut her wrist with the razor, bleeding all over the project on her desk.

After Jenny was hospitalized, she continued in treatment and gradually learned to set limits with her coworkers and family. She insisted on a contract that clearly defined her job and her hours. She turned away any requests that did not fall within this description. As she regained control of her life, her confidence grew and she learned to value herself without always having to please others. The urge to cut herself returned from time to time, but then finally faded away forever.

When your personal boundaries are well-developed, they no longer have to be defended by desperate actions. When the outlines of yourself are well-defined, then within them can grow an enduring sense of wholeness, peace, and security.

When Sara left my office and began driving home, as we later discovered, she suddenly turned and headed for the highway. She drove as if in a trance, making turns intuitively without knowing her destination. She rolled down the highway for nearly two hours until the car finally turned onto an exit ramp. As dusk fell she found herself in front of the cemetery.

Sara faced row upon row of similar looking headstones. The length of the cemetery seemed boundless. She began walking amid the stones looking for a landmark until she was nearly at the center of the graveyard, surrounded by rows of tombstones that stretched as far as she could see in all directions.

Sara broke into a run. She zigzagged among the stones, searching frantically until she arrived at a small headstone that bore her family's name. She stood panting by her father's grave and felt herself filling with rage.

Who was this man she once thought loved her so much? How could he have even thought about hurting her? How could he have subjected her to such terror or so brutalized her mother? And how dare he die before she could confront him and get her questions answered.

Sara kicked the ground over her father's grave and began beating her fists on the headstone until they were raw and bloodied. She never felt the pain. When she finally stopped, she was overcome with fatigue and fell asleep in the grass.

When Sara came back to her senses, she was just a few blocks from her house. She had just filled the gas tank that day, but it was nearly empty. It was two in the morning when she pulled into the driveway. Jonathan was frantic with worry and had already called my office and the police. When he saw her drive up, he was relieved. But when she appeared bedraggled, her clothes covered with dirt and stained with grass, her hands swollen and bloody, he felt alarmed and outraged.

Sara could not remember where she had been. The last thing she remembered was leaving my office. She had been upset by something during the session, but she could not remember what it was. She looked for reassurance in Jonathan's face, but when she met his gaze, all she could see was anger and suspicion and she felt terrified. She felt as though her world was crumbling all around her.

Sara slept that night in Megan's room, clinging to her like a stuffed toy. That night the nightmare came back. But this time she was an observer, watching the child running frightened in the forest, and she noticed for the first time that it was a little boy.

9

Impulse
Filling up an Empty Shell

Just try to explain to anyone the art of fasting!
Anyone who has no feeling for it cannot be made to
understand it.

"A HUNGER ARTIST"
FRANZ KAFKA

The extreme emotions of the person with BPD are matched by her extreme behaviors. She may deprive herself to the point of starvation or may indulge to drastic excess. These shifting compulsions contribute to the discontinuity of her identity, leaving a chameleon-like impression.

The arena of behavior covers the range of human appetites and may include food, sex, and aggression, as well as acquiring possessions, using alcohol and drugs, and the excitement of taking risks. If you are borderline, you are likely to indulge in more than one of these areas. They may become interchangeable so that measures to suppress one kind of behavior results in the prompt emergence of another.

Sylvia was a twenty-seven-year-old restaurant manager who was admitted to the hospital because of severe bulimia. She had been binging and purging several times a day. Upon entering the hospital, she was prevented from vomiting by constant observation for two hours after each meal. On the fourth day in the hospital, she began to make cuts up and down the length of her forearms, using a razor blade she had smuggled in. This act of aggression toward herself discharged the tension that was usually relieved by vomiting.

The impulsive behaviors in BPD all have common elements. They are immediately gratifying and are preceded by a building of tension, which the impulsive act relieves. They are usually risky, and there is little concern for negative consequences in the future. They are often ritualized, with a stereotypical pattern from one time to the next. They may seem irresistible, with tension mounting to an intolerable degree if the act does not occur. They are frequently followed by feelings of regret or remorse.

These behaviors are truly mood-altering. They are intended to put an end to feelings of emptiness and despair. And some may also seek to establish a fragment of identity.

I Am What I Eat

In bulimia, vast quantities of food may be eaten at a single sitting followed by self-induced vomiting. Laxatives may also be used in a vain attempt to purge the body of what has been taken in. This behavior often accompanies severe dieting, with the binge occurring as a response to extreme hunger and the purge intended to restore weight control.

Once a binge has been triggered, appetite becomes insatiable, with eating limited only by extreme physical distress. Vomiting relieves this distress and completes the cycle.

While bulimia may occur alone, many bulimics engage in other compulsive behaviors such as shoplifting and drug abuse. For many, bulimia is only one manifestation of BPD.

The binge is a response to extreme feelings of emptiness, both physical and emotional. The attempt to get filled up may have other overtones as well. The mouth is an instrument not only for feeding, but for aggression and sexuality. When we speak of "biting someone's head off" or "chewing them out," we reflect the aggression inherent in eating.

Purging may also contain symbolic meaning. The word "purge" means both to empty and to cleanse or purify. Purging may be an attempt to get rid of what is impure or evil. For some, it may be an attempt to undo sexual acts that have been unacceptable. Purging is another sign of a fragmented self-concept, in which a part of the self can be sacrificed to save the rest.

Anorexia nervosa is self-imposed starvation that results in unnatural thinness. It is the ultimate act of self-deprivation. The quest for thinness may become the anorexic's dominant identifying feature. This overconcern with body image reflects the fragility of the anorexic's identity.

Both bulimia and anorexia are struggles for control. Many people with eating disorders, like people with BPD, have had their bodies violated by others. People with anorexia control absolutely what goes into their bodies. People with bulimia attempt to control what stays in. Both struggle to control their body size, a single measurable dimension of self-worth.

People with anorexia fear losing control of their appetites and becoming obese. Some have been overweight at some time in their lives; for others this fear is unfounded. They may see themselves as obese even when already painfully emaciated. This may be a reflection of how they imagine they would look if they gave their appetites full rein.

For those with BPD, anorexia nervosa is another example of the inability to modulate feelings. The only way to deal with feeling insatiable is to turn off hunger altogether. In many religions, sacrifice and self-denial are expressions of atonement. With anorexia nervosa, fasting is often brought on by guilt and, like purging, is a way to feel cleansed of sin.

I Am Who Loves Me

Sex may serve to provide momentary pleasure, a refuge from loneliness and boredom, and a prop for sagging self-esteem.

Through splitting, a person's lover may be seen as a shining hero so that she may bask in his glow. Later, both may be condemned together.

If you are borderline, your feelings about sexuality are likely full of contradictions. Especially if you have been abused, sex may be frightening and laden with guilt. But it may also be the only way you know to be touched and valued. It may be your only apparent means of power over others in the face of overwhelming feelings of powerlessness. You may strive to be attractive through dieting and dressing up while at the same time feel guilty for your sexual urges.

People who have been abused are often revictimized again and again. Reliving victimization may be a way of trying to control it, justify it, or avenge it. Becoming the seducer turns the tables on the balance of power, even if it is only an illusion. Repeated sexual conquests reconfirm the weakness and treachery of all men, softening your own feelings of worthlessness and guilt. At the same time, seductive behavior may be the acid test in your search for the honest man, the good parent who will never willfully betray you.

Sexual abstinence may defend against strong sexual urges. This may be reinforced by special means. For example, excessive dieting may go beyond the point of sexual attractiveness to emaciation and loss of all sexual characteristics, a turnoff for most would-be lovers. Joining a strict religious order or cult may be another way of gaining support for self-control while at the same time acquiring a group identity.

Both excessive indulgence in sexuality and abstinence from it serve also to avoid the intimacy that develops in a balanced love relationship.

I Am What I Own

Shoplifting and compulsive shopping both involve acquiring property. Both also frequently focus on clothing and other bodily adornments.

In the movie *Back to the Future*, the hero returns to the 1950s wearing Calvin Klein jeans. Everyone naturally assumes his name is Calvin. Why would anyone emblazon someone else's name on his hip pocket? Today, such fashion symbols have an enormous influence on self-esteem for many people. If you are borderline, wearing the right things may be an important part of your identity. It may also be another way to feel cared for and loved.

Both shoplifters and compulsive spenders "live on the edge," risking getting caught or going deeply into debt. Risky behavior helps relieve feelings of emptiness and boredom. Both may feel entitled to have the things they acquire. Both also may victimize others, since spending money can be an effective way to get back at an uncaring parent or spouse.

Like other compulsions, the satisfaction is short-lived and may end in disappointment and guilt, if not financial ruin or imprisonment.

I Am What I Drink or Smoke

Alcohol and drug abuse provide a rapid and effective way to alter mood. Uppers elevate mood, while downers numb all feeling. As with other compulsions, substance abuse is an attempt to escape from intolerable feelings such as helplessness and worthlessness, loneliness, emptiness, and boredom. As with other compulsions, its effects are incomplete and fleeting.

When substance abuse occurs in a group, it may provide an instant bond with other group members, creating a sense of identity within the group. It may even create links with other family members who have been role models for substance abuse. If you are borderline, parental abuse of alcohol and drugs may have set up the fundamental conditions of your world as a child.

Substance abuse is a particularly insidious problem since it may cloud thinking and set the scene for activating other compulsions. If you are to regain control and to heal, it is crucially important to have a clear mind.

Substance abuse also contributes to the fragmentation of experience. Intoxication removes us from the normal flow of consciousness. The memory of what occurs while intoxicated may be lacking in clarity and completeness. We may also disavow full responsibility for behavior that occurs under the influence of substances, as if someone else had committed the acts.

All of the compulsive behaviors described above are outgrowths of the discontinuity of experience, emotions, and identity that is typical of BPD. They reflect the splitting of perceptions of self and others into extremes of good and evil that can be magically separated from each other by symbolic acts.

Self-mutilation is another manifestation of this discontinuity. It deserves a separate chapter because of its dramatic impact both on the person with BPD and those around her, because it provides a unique window for examining and understanding her inner life, and because of its strong association with BPD.

*S*ara called the next day, distraught and tearful, and we arranged an extra session. While she usually came to the office dressed in frilly and often revealing clothes and was meticulously made up, this time she arrived in a baggy sweatshirt and jeans, her hair unwashed and pulled tightly back in a ponytail, dark circles under her eyes. She recalled very little of the previous day, only that she had arrived home in the middle of the night and Jonathan had been angry. She had apparently driven a long way. This was the second time she had driven somewhere and could not remember where she had gone. We were to learn much later where these flights had taken her.

Sara did not ask and I did not volunteer the contents of our previous session. I assumed that she was not yet ready to face the horrifying memories that had been uncovered. Her emotional defenses now protected her from them once more. She recounted the dream about the fleeing child and felt oddly guilty, but could not explain why. She digressed quickly from the dream content to her irritation with her older daughter Lisa, who was lately picking on Megan unmercifully. This seemed a trivial subject, given how upset she had been about the previous day, but she warmed quickly to it, insisting that Lisa was turning into a very naughty little girl.

Sara called to cancel her next session, rescheduling for the following week, but then missed that session as well. Jonathan called to voice concerns about her behavior and I saw them together the next day. Sara had been staying out late with some regularity and had been drinking. When she drank, she became hostile and defensive. They were arguing nightly and Sara was now sleeping with Megan all the time. He was most concerned, however, about her attitude toward Lisa, which had changed drastically. She always seemed angry at the child and screamed at her frequently over trivial offenses. Lisa had begun to cling to Jonathan whenever Sara was around.

When I expressed my concern about Sara's relapsing alcohol abuse, she became indignant. "Whose side are you on, anyway?" she screamed, "I thought you were supposed to be my doctor, not Jonathan's!" Sara acknowledged punishing Lisa, but she insisted that Lisa deserved any punishment she got; she was really turning into an impossible child.

Sara came late to the next several sessions. She was sullen and lacking in her usual spontaneity. There was a remarkable variety in her appearance at these sessions, one day appearing in dissheveled work clothes, another in a dark business suit, and yet another in a tight-fitting minidress that became even more revealing as she slouched carelessly in her chair. I felt, during that session, as if I were being challenged by a defiant and provocative adolescent.

Sara continued to drink. It became apparent that she was frequenting bars and sometimes picking up men, but she would stop short of going to bed with them, reveling in their frustration and anger. This continued until one night when she was badly beaten.

10

Rescuing the Angel Within

Understanding Self-Mutilation

And if thy right eye offend thee, pluck it out and cast it from thee: for it is profitable for thee that one of thy members shall perish, and not that thy whole body shall be cast into Hell.

MATTHEW 5:29

Perhaps the most shocking and mysterious of all borderline behaviors is self-mutilation. It is virtually a trademark for BPD although it sometimes occurs in other conditions.

Self-mutilation may be as simple as superficial scratches on the skin with fingernails or a blunt instrument, or as tragic and complicated as the surgical excision of a body part. Some injuries are visible to all while others are well hidden. Some are inflicted with elaborate ritual, while others convey special meaning that can be deciphered by the knowledgeable observer like the hieroglyphics in an ancient tomb. These injuries are often mistaken for suicide attempts.

Whether burns or cuts or penetrating wounds, these self-inflicted injuries are the products of compulsion. Like other compulsions, a buildup of tension leads to an irresistible urge, and the tension is discharged by the act.

Self-injury brings horror to the hearts of family members. They may also view it with anger as a form of defiance. Because it presents serious risk to health and life, it may become the occasion for an involuntary hospitalization. Extreme measures, such as constant observation or physical restraint, may be brought to bear to prevent the more serious forms of self-injury. The power struggle that follows may become one of the forces that keeps the compulsion alive.

To the borderline person, self-mutilation may be rich in meaning.

Self-Mutilation as Punishment

This is perhaps the simplest interpretation of self-mutilation. If you are borderline, you may be filled with guilt over real and imagined crimes. Self-mutilation may be a particularly fitting punishment for the crime of forbidden sexuality. The origins of guilt may relate to present-day relationships and behaviors or may be connected with early childhood experiences, such as incest. In the myth of Oedipus, Oedipus is overwhelmed with guilt upon discovering that he has unknowingly killed his father and married his mother. He punishes himself by putting out his eyes.

Self-Mutilation as Sacrifice

Through splitting, a body part or the body as whole may come to symbolize all that is bad about the self. The body may, therefore, be made a kind of scapegoat to be punished for the sins of its owner. This was the case for Tony, a twenty-year-old man who punished himself for lustful thoughts by taking literally the biblical injunction quoted at the beginning of this chapter. He maintained that it was "better to lose an eye than to burn in hell." After losing the eye, he claimed that he no longer had lustful thoughts. He believed, even a year later, that he had changed his life for the better by destroying his eye.

Tony's sacrifice drastically altered his identity. His symbolic rebirth set the first part of his life apart from the second in a dramatic example of the discontinuity that marks the life of a person with BPD.

Sacrifice has been a part of man's rituals for protecting himself since the beginning of history. The letting of blood is a frequent element of sacrificial ritual and appears as well in the self-mutilative acts of the borderline person. Such sacrifice may also be experienced as purification.

Self-Mutilation as a Cry for Help

The more visible forms of self-mutilation effectively rivet the attention of others and invite rescue. A common outcome is hospitalization, which may be outwardly feared but secretly longed for. If you are borderline, this may be particularly true when you feel out of control and in need of the structured environment of the hospital. Being hospitalized may, at times, be a means of drawing others into closer involvement with you and, at other times, may be a way of escaping from relationships that have become too close and threatening.

Self-Mutilation as Directed Pain

Sometimes emotional pain seems impossible to bear. If you are borderline, self-inflicted physical pain may serve as distraction from intolerable emotional distress. It may also show others an unmistakeable sign that you are hurt.

In the face of intolerable emotional pain, you may instead retreat into a numbed or unfeeling state. After a time, this too becomes intolerable, and self-injury may become a means for renewing contact with the world of sensation. At times, the emotionally numb state may extend to physical anesthesia, so that severe injuries may be inflicted with a minimum of pain.

Self-Mutilation as Coded Message

The specific type of self-mutilation may contain within it a symbolic message to yourself or others. For example, the casting away of an eye is a symbolic renunciation of looking at forbidden things. This was true for Gretchen, a young woman who carefully cut a large "X" on the lower part of her abdomen. She would rework the wound with each stressful situation, leaving a permanent scar on her body. This universally understood sign presented a clear and forbidding message to any would-be lover that that part of her body was off limits.

Self-Mutilation as Reenactment

Since most people with BPD have experienced physical or sexual abuse, self-abuse may represent a reenactment of the earlier injury. This compulsion to repeat earlier traumatic events has been recognized since Freud and may represent an unconscious attempt to create a new, happier ending to a painful memory. Repeating painful experiences may also be a way of developing emotional continuity between past and present.

Borderline people may also provoke a reenactment of their victimization at the hands of others. In a particularly curious variation of this, known in medicine as Munchausen's syndrome, patients will go from hospital to hospital with falsified evidence of serious physical illness and undergo operation after operation at the hands of unwitting doctors. Getting others to inflict the wounds may be viewed as indirect self-mutilation.

Whatever its particular meaning for each individual, self-mutilation presents the most significant risk and hindrance to therapy, short of suicide. Psychotherapy with a patient who self-mutilates is like digging for precious artifacts in the midst of a minefield. The work is often painstaking and intense. Suicide can abruptly reduce the entire project to rubble.

Sara was found wandering, dazed and battered, by the police and taken to the emergency room of the county medical hospital. She was admitted overnight to treat her injuries, none of which turned out to be serious. As soon as she was considered medically stable, I arranged for her transfer to the psychiatric hospital for further treatment of her alcohol addiction and the self-defeating behavior that was associated with it.

As Sara went through the detoxification stage of her treatment and her thinking became clearer, she was overcome with remorse about her recent escapades. She remained in considerable pain for several days from her injuries, but refused even aspirin to treat it.

"I got what I deserved," she told me on her third day in the hospital. "Besides, I've been numb so long from drinking it's a relief to feel anything again." She hated herself for how she had treated Jonathan and was too embarrassed to face him. She hoped he would never have to find out how she had set herself up for the beating. She asked him not to visit until she was feeling better.

On the seventh day, Sara awoke in the middle of the night panic-stricken. She had dreamed that Jonathan had shot himself to death. The dream had seemed so real that she could not be reassured that he was all right and insisted on calling him then and there. She asked him to visit the next day with the children. He had felt confused by the way she seemed to be shutting him out and received the invitation with relief and renewed hope.

When we met the next day, I remarked to Sara that this was not the first time that she had avoided someone she loved in order to protect a secret. She recalled her self-imposed exile from her father's presence and the untimely death that had prevented her repatriation forever, and for the first time since his death she wept for him. In her reenactment of these events with Jonathan, she had brought them to the same conclusion in her imagination. Fortunately, this time she would be given a second chance.

Within the safety of the hospital, Sara was able to recover the *childhood memories that we had briefly uncovered earlier in treatment. This occurred at first by way of flashbacks, first to her own recent beating, then to the images of her mother's beatings at the hands of her father. The flashbacks occurred without warning and with a vividness that erased the intervening years.*

"Whack! Whack!" The sounds followed her around for days, interrupting her sleep and intruding upon our sessions until she wanted desperately to run away. But this time the hospital doors stood firmly in her way. She began thinking about ways to kill herself, insisting that everyone would be better off without her. She wished that she had a gun so that she could do the job properly. Then she remembered the gun that her father had held so many times to her head and the moment of relief that she felt when the gun came away, followed moments later by her mommy's sobs of pain. And she felt deeply ashamed.

Sara learned that the close connection between her own escape from danger and her mother's pain as these scenes ended left her confused and ashamed of her feelings. She remembered wishing each time that the gun would go away and feeling guilty later that the answer to her prayer brought her mother such pain. She could not have known then that her mother had prayed for the same endings, gladly accepting the beatings as long as her baby was safe.

Sara struggled with her shame and guilt. She learned that her fantasy about shooting herself was her symbolic way of undoing the ending of the childhood scene. She learned that sacrificing herself in this way now would not spare her mother, but only bring her more pain.

Sara became able to look back at herself as a small and frightened four-year-old child and to forgive that child for her helplessness and terror. She understood for the first time that she was as helpless a victim as her mother and was not responsible for the outcome. Then the flashbacks subsided and stopped. For a while, Sara felt at peace.

11

Suicide

Dying Without Death

I have met the enemy and he is us.
POGO
WALT KELLY

S uicide is the ultimate expression of black-and-white thinking. Most people with BPD think about suicide. Many threaten it. Some attempt it. A few complete it.

About one in ten people with BPD die by suicide. This most often occurs early in treatment or in the absence of treatment. Those who die are often among the most productive individuals who had very high expectations of themselves. Relief from their anguish may have been just around the corner, but they could not wait.

Suicide is a response to intolerable pain that appears to have no end. When chosen, it feels like the only possible way out of pain. Suicidal people feel hopeless and helpless. They are wounded emotionally and cannot envision healing or surviving for as long as healing would take.

For people with BPD, these feelings of hopelessness and helplessness often occur on the heels of a rejection or personal failure. Rejection feels absolute and permanent, leaving them feeling unlovable and imagining a lifetime of unbearable loneliness.

Suicide may also be a surrender to overwhelming responsibility. In the black-and-white world of BPD, self-imposed standards of responsibility may be extreme. Suicide is a final abdication of responsibility. It is the choice of "none" when "all" is impossible.

Suicide may be an answer to an impossible dilemma. It may be the only apparent way out of an abusive relationship for someone who is terrified of being alone. It may be the only apparent solution to a situation that demands giving up something that is precious.

The common thread is the inability to see through the fog of the moment's crisis. The suicidal person is in pain now and is unable to draw on the past or future for consolation or hope. This discontinuity is a hallmark of being borderline. No wonder so many people with BPD consider suicide!

Donald was a thirty-seven-year-old executive in the midst of a marital separation that he had initiated after falling in love with another woman. As the separation evolved toward divorce, Donald became overwhelmed with guilt over the effect of the decision on his three small children. When he spoke of leaving them, tears came to his eyes as he imagined their pain.

Donald was unwilling to give up his lover and the comfort she brought him. He was equally unable to live with his decision to divorce, which he considered abandoning his family. Seeing no other choices, he took an overdose of drugs.

As he recovered from the suicide attempt, it was pointed out to him how much more painful his death would have been to his children than the divorce. He replied that he would not have been around to endure the guilt. Such an intensely selfish response was a strange paradox in a man so strongly motivated by compassion.

Hopelessness and helplessness are also part of the syndrome called depression. Together with disturbances of sleep, appetite, energy level, and motivation, they mark the presence of biological changes that may seriously warp one's outlook. These biological events may follow adverse life circumstances, may occur out of the blue, or may result from an underlying physical problem, such as thyroid disease or the effects of certain medications.

I once saw, in consultation, an elderly man who was hospitalized with tuberculosis. When I first saw him, he was deep in despair. He told me that he had a horrible, incurable disease. What's more, he had been burdened for ten years with the care of his wife, who had crippling arthritis. He denied having any hobby or interest. He was waiting to die.

I found among his medications one that is well known to cause depression. I withheld that drug and returned two days later. I was greeted warmly by a man who appeared at least ten years younger. He was bright and energetic. I reinterviewed him from the beginning. He told me he was recovering well from tuberculosis, which he understood to be curable. He talked about the companionship of his beloved wife and the joy and comfort she brought him. He described an extensive wood shop that kept him busy and productive in his retirement. He talked of travel plans and other activities he looked forward to. He was content.

The rapid change in perspective occurred as a result of a chemical change in the man's brain. The circumstances of his life otherwise had not changed. Only the emphasis was altered.

One of life's most reliable conditions is its unpredictability. I am reminded of a character in a movie who had just lost all that he valued. When asked why he didn't kill himself, he replied, "I'm too curious to find out what's going to happen next." To a person with the fragmented outlook of BPD, looking beyond the present with an open mind is inconceivable.

Suicide is not caused merely by a wish to die. It is a symbolic act rich in meaning and highly individual. While for some it is primarily an expression of hopelessness and despair, for others it reflects intolerable rage or guilt.

Suicide is the ultimate means to control destiny when life feels out of control. Little in life is more mysterious and uncontrollable than how we will die. Suicide enables us not only to choose the means but to select the time of our deaths. It is like suddenly standing face-to-face with an armed intruder who has been secretly stalking us, taking the gun, and pointing it at our own head. The danger remains, but the stalker is disarmed and powerless.

Like self-mutilation and fasting, suicide can also be a sacrifice. The suicidal person may believe that others would be better off without her. She may feel that she has been a burden to others or consider life insurance or other possible financial advantages that her death would bring her family. She may overlook her dreadful legacy to survivors—grieving for a loved one who chose death over them.

Suicide is an often hateful act. It is a willful abandonment of others. It is a message to others that they have failed disastrously and irrevocably. It is playing out a childish fantasy of revenge: "You'll be sorry when I'm dead!"

Consider Julia, a middle-aged wife and mother of four, who prepared a roast, set the oven timer, and left a note that said "good-bye" and "dinner is ready" before taking a fatal overdose in the bedroom.

Consider Tanya, who blew her brains out while talking to her mother on the telephone.

Consider Sharon, who asphyxiated herself with the exhaust fumes from her husband's new sports car.

These women all left unforgettable messages for their survivors. "See how I've sacrificed for you all my life and even now." "See how you've failed me." "How dare you value anything more than me!" These messages were a lasting punishment for those left behind.

Some seek suicide as liberation from torment. It is common for deeply depressed people to show a sudden elevation of mood once the decision to die has been made. They can appear peaceful and content. At such times, hospital staff may judge a patient to be better and remove some of the safeguards against suicide, which may then come as a surprise. These people are determined, and their suicidal acts are lethal.

Many imagine suicide as a reunion with the dead. Our tendency to idealize the dead is strong. With the black-and-white thinking of BPD, this tendency is even stronger. At times of despair, fantasies of reunion with lost loved ones may be compelling, and suicide is a response to such fantasies. The longing for reunion may be symbolized by the choice of suicide method, which may resemble a particular person's mode of death, or may mimic it precisely if that person also died by suicide. Examples of other clues to these fantasies include the decision to die on the anniversary of another's death or while wearing an article of clothing or jewelry that belonged to that person.

Suicide is often ambivalent. Most suicidal acts allow for some chance of rescue. They resemble Russian roulette. Death may be attractive enough to flirt with, but its permanence is much harder to embrace.

Suicide is a fantasy of dying without death. It is a chance to seek the love and devotion in death that was so elusive in life. It is the fantasy of attending our own funerals, like Tom Sawyer, and seeing how we are grieved. It is an opportunity for revenge, but we cannot savor revenge in death just as surely as we are not required to endure the guilt over the havoc we have wreaked.

Suicide is an enduring legacy. Survivors are scarred for life. Children experience horrible rejection, abandonment, guilt, and rage as they personalize a parent's suicide. Their security and trust is shaken to its foundations. Their sense of order is turned upside down. Something unthinkable has happened. The world has turned into a treacherous place. For most adults and children, suicide is strictly forbidden. When the taboo is breached successfully by someone close, it is lifted forever. Suicide becomes simply one of the options for escaping pain. If you kill yourself, your children become many times more likely to eventually end their lives the same way. Suicide is a wound that time can never heal completely.

Suicide is power over others. The person who threatens suicide is like a terrorist who straps dynamite to his body. He takes hostages. He gets everyone's attention. He makes demands. "Prove that you love me." "Make my life worthwhile," or simply, "Don't go away." The effects of such blackmail are invariably destructive. If the demands are satisfied, the threats are very likely to be repeated whenever frustration occurs. Any gains are illusory. The lover who refrains from breaking up a relationship because of a suicide threat remains a prisoner who will look for escape at the earliest opportunity.

Rodney was a twenty-six-year-old alcoholic who had been married for eight years to Cheryl. Rodney beat Cheryl regularly throughout most of their relationship. Cheryl had made several attempts to leave and had been drawn back sometimes by promises and sometimes by threats. She finally found her way to a women's shelter and hired an attorney. At that point, Rodney shot himself in the abdomen with a small caliber handgun.

When Rodney regained consciousness in the surgical intensive care unit, Cheryl was by his bedside, flowers in hand, promising never to leave him again. She was momentarily overcome by guilt that would later give way to rage as the cycle of abuse and promises resumed. Rodney and Cheryl were both borderline.

The short-term gratification of successful blackmail not only reinforced Rodney's tendency to become self-destructive at times of desperation, but also undermined any motivation he might have had to seek treatment designed to change his behavior. But emotional pain cannot always be so easily escaped.

Eventually self-destructive behavior adds to the burden of being borderline and pain becomes overwhelming. Changing behavior is the only permanent solution to the pain. Treatment is the tool to bring about that change.

When Sara came home from the hospital, Jonathan welcomed her with open arms. He was glad to see her sober and strong. He never questioned any of the behavior that led up to the assault and her hospitalization. There was no reproach.

At first, Sara was grateful for Jonathan's unconditional love. She felt secure and invested her time and energy in her recovery program. She attended Alcoholics Anonymous meetings daily and worked the Twelve Steps, which form the foundation of the program.

Several months later, at the peak of Sara's serenity, they went on vacation to the beach. This was where she had always felt most at peace. She loved to listen to the rhythm of the waves rolling in and crashing on the shore. She loved to run along the water's edge and still delighted in playing in the surf.

As soon as they had spread out their beach towels, Sara kicked off her sandals, pulled off her cover-up and ran into the water. Jonathan and the children followed. Sara looked back and smiled as she watched them splashing each other by the water's edge.

Sara watched as Jonathan lifted Lisa high over his head, dunked her in the water and pulled the squealing child out again. Then suddenly she panicked. She could not see Megan anywhere. She called out to Jonathan but he could not hear her over the sound of the surf. She headed toward them, her heart thumping so loudly she could no longer hear the waves. She felt as if everything around her had stopped and she was moving in slow motion.

As she watched, Jonathan again hoisted a child aloft. Sara saw with relief that it was Megan. But the relief was only momentary. Her heart still pounded wildly and she could feel herself getting sick to her stomach. When she finally reached her unsuspecting family, still frolicking in the water, she told

Jonathan abruptly that she had to leave. She ran up the beach, hurriedly packed their belongings, and headed for the car. Jonathan and the children followed obediently, disappointed that their fun was so inexplicably cut short.

As they drove back to the cottage, Sara blasted Jonathan verbally. How could he have been so careless? Didn't he realize Megan might have drowned? How could he have endangered her so? Jonathan had perceived no danger. Megan had always been right by his side, safe and sound. Sara could not be reassured. And she would not return to the beach. At her insistence, they drove home that night.

When Sara reached home exhausted, she fell asleep and once again found herself in the forest, searching for a lost child. This time when she looked at the child, it was Megan.

12

Being in Treatment

I begin to see. Today I am not all wood.
ANN SEXTON

Individual therapy is the cornerstone of treatment for BPD. Treatment begins with choosing a therapist. Selecting a competent and compatible therapist is crucial, since successful treatment depends on developing a trusting and mutually respectful alliance between your therapist and you.

Therapy is an active partnership. It is not "done to you" like a surgical procedure, but is a cooperative investigation of your emotional life. You and your therapist share responsibility for the outcome. Your therapist must provide a safe and caring environment for talking about your feelings. You must be willing to be open and honest about all aspects of your emotional life.

The principal goal of treatment is to develop a stable sense of identity with an enduring set of values and beliefs. From this accomplishment comes a sense of continuity that makes it possible to weather momentary misfortune and distress while maintaining hope. When you can tolerate painful feelings, you will no longer need to flee from pain in impulsive self-defeating ways.

Your Relationship with Your Therapist

The relationship you develop with your therapist is likely to become as charged with emotion as any of your other important relationships. You bring your borderline defenses and coping strategies with you into treatment.

You will, at times, idealize your therapist. At other times, you will perceive betrayal and wish to flee. Such splitting presents the most common obstacle to completing treatment. It is indeed common for people with BPD to reenact the fragility of their relationships by engaging in many brief episodes of treatment with various therapists. Anticipating disillusionment may help you to endure it long enough to finish treatment.

Another serious risk in treatment is the potential for revictimization. Therapy is not immune to your tendency to reenact early trauma. In fact, treatment provides a real chance to change the ending of the early trauma when the therapist maintains trust and remains caring and respectful. While most therapists are ethical and responsible and are equal to the task of maintaining proper boundaries, a few are not.

How can you judge your therapist objectively so that you can avoid ending good treatment prematurely but still be alert to the possibility of inappropriate treatment in unethical hands?

A therapist's only legitimate compensation for treatment is the fee he or she receives for treating you. If your therapist seeks any other personal gain or self-gratification through your treatment, then your trust has been violated. This goes especially for any sexual contact with you. Regardless of how it may come about, any sexual intimacy between a therapist and a patient is unethical and is certain to bring you further emotional harm.

Some of the same principles that apply to protecting children from abuse apply to protecting yourself in therapy. If it doesn't feel okay, it probably isn't. If you are threatened or sworn to secrecy, you have almost certainly been violated.

If you are uncomfortable or uncertain about what is happening in treatment, consultation with another therapist may be helpful. You may request a referral from your therapist or find a consultant on your own. Consultation can help clarify misperceptions and resolve impasses in otherwise sound treatment. Most therapists are receptive to this strategy.

If your therapist tries to discourage you from consultation, or refuses it altogether, watch out! It is important that you feel free when talking with a consultant to disclose any aspect of your treatment.

Your Therapist's Relationship with You

Because of your special vulnerability, your therapist holds considerable power in your relationship. With this power goes an equally awesome responsibility to live up to your trust. This responsibility can be draining.

Therapy creates powerful emotions, both for patient and therapist. A good therapist is always listening "with a third ear" for indirect messages about his patient's feelings about him. It is too easy, for example, for a therapist listening to a patient raging with anger at a family member or coworker to join with the patient's anger and miss seeing that she is really angry at him.

A therapist can also be tuned so exquisitely into the nuances of a patient's feelings as to be virtually paralyzed to intervene. With some patients, I have been aware at times of feeling held in suspense in their presence. My breathing becomes shallow and my voice very quiet as if I fear being noticed at all by my patient. This feeling invariably has occurred with patients who have been severely abused, and whom I perceived as being particularly wounded and fragile. At such times, I have been struck by how this feeling might resemble that of a frightened child avoiding the notice of her abuser. In this way, my patients have unwittingly taught me how it feels to be them.

Sometimes, it feels as if nothing I can ever say or do will please my patient. Sometimes it feels as if displeasing her in any way will bring retaliation. These reactions are lessons about my patients' experiences as children who were made to feel that they could never do anything right or who were always singled out for punishment.

Patients often make threats that place therapists in horrible dilemmas. When a patient appears to be in real danger of committing suicide, for example, but absolutely refuses hospitalization, the therapist faces the choice between risking his patient's life or forcing her to be hospitalized. The therapist risks being seen as abandoning her on the one hand or imprisoning her on the other.

Chantelle was a twenty-three-year-old woman, married only six months, who was feeling panicked at the sudden onslaught of sexual demands from her new husband. She came to treatment as a result of her refusal to eat and a weight loss of thirty pounds since her wedding day. Her husband felt mystified and helpless. As she became more and more emaciated, he withdrew his sexual advances.

During her third treatment session, she disclosed that she had bought some razor blades and was thinking about killing herself. "You can't stop me," she told her doctor, "and if you try, I'll surely kill myself once I get the chance." To make matters worse, she told her husband that if he allowed the doctor to put her in the hospital, she would never forgive him. The husband, already feeling guilty over his wife's desperate state of mind, promised to watch her night and day in order to keep her from having to go to the hospital.

Chantelle saw her doctor as a powerful authority figure who was threatening to lock her up. What she did not see was that her doctor was as much a captive as she, held hostage by her threats of suicide. Rather than a willful display of power, his insistence upon hospitalization was a natural outcome of his responsibility to protect her.

Leaving a Trail

As your relationship with your therapist unfolds and deepens, you are likely to experience feelings that you find too painful or embarrassing to express directly. These may include feelings of love and gratitude, as well as feelings of anger and resentment.

You may wish that your therapist hold and comfort you and may even find yourself fantasizing about making love together. You may also have vengeful fantasies of attacking your therapist physically or emotionally, or of some terrible accident destroying him.

When feelings, such as simultaneous love and murderous rage, are too painful to bear, you may not even be fully aware of them yourself. You will undoubtedly leave trails, however, that both you and your therapist, if you are astute detectives, can use to discover these feelings and their origins. Some signposts of hidden feelings may appear directly in the way you deal with therapy.

You may become silent and withhold all your thoughts and feelings from your therapist's scrutiny. The quality of your silence may be dark and threatening and fill the room with tension. Or it may be aloof and indifferent, shutting him out of your emotional life altogether.

You may arrive at your sessions late or miss them altogether. This both avoids any need to confront your feelings and provokes a distracting confrontation between you and your therapist over how these indiscretions are to be managed. The real limits of the relationship, including time limits and fees, which usually form the background for the action, become thrust into the limelight.

You may withhold payment for your sessions. This tells your therapist indirectly that you do not value his services and deprives him of his livelihood. It may also reflect the wish that your therapist provide unlimited love and nurturing without requiring anything in return. You may also express this wish by making demands on your therapist outside the usual boundaries of your relationship. This may include demands during sessions, such as requests for touching and holding, and after-hours calls.

The after-hours call makes a special claim on your therapist's life and loyalty. It reaches into the privacy of his home and asks for a piece of time that has been set aside to meet his own needs. Therapists, like others, need time for rest and recreation, personal errands, reading and learning, privacy and intimacy. They need time to be with their families and to nurture their personal relationships.

Therapists understand that emergencies occur and are prepared for an occasional demand on their personal time, but when these intrusions become frequent, they are likely to feel frustrated and resentful. These feelings may interfere with your therapist's ability to treat you.

The urge to call your therapist may have many roots. You may feel the need to confirm his existence beyond the narrow confines of your sessions. Just as other aspects of your life lack constancy, you may feel that people cease to exist when they are no longer with you. You may be trying to define the limits of the relationship, if these have not been clearly spelled out from the start, or to test the consistency of the limits. You may be looking for proof that your therapist really cares, or perhaps for confirmation that he is just as fake as others who have betrayed your trust.

Calling your therapist may become a compulsion, interchangeable with other compulsions that help temporarily to relieve emotional tension, fill up the emptiness inside, and restore contact with the real world.

Other emotional signposts may appear in the way you handle your life outside of therapy. You may turn angry feelings toward your therapist into self-destructive impulses, such as increasing the frequency of eating binges, or mutilating yourself. You may act out feeling deprived or frustrated by compulsive spending or shoplifting. You may act on sexual urges by having an affair or going from lover to lover.

Suicide threats, gestures, or attempts are a particularly

destructive way to act out painful feelings. A suicide gesture is a token attempt in which the chosen method is clearly nonlethal or the opportunity for rescue was clearly arranged. Rather than attempts to die, gestures are messages to others, including therapists. Unfortunately, even gestures can be miscalculated, and sometimes turn lethal.

Threatening suicide is a sure way to get your therapist's attention. Coupled with the after-hours phone call, it is a powerful weapon that can threaten your therapist's security and damage his ability to help you. Suicide threats also provoke confrontation, as it did for Deidre.

My telephone rang and there was a long silence at the other end. Finally, Deidre's childlike voice said very softly, "I'm okay." I asked what was wrong, and there was more silence, then, "Really . . . I'm okay."

This was Deidre's standard way of signalling extreme distress. Suicidal hints soon followed. "Don't worry, I haven't done anything yet." This meant, "Worry plenty, but I won't let you do anything about it."

Deidre would next ask me to promise not to hospitalize her despite her obvious danger. What's more, she would tell me a host of reasons why she could not be hospitalized, including the unavailability of anyone to care for her young children, and other compelling obligations or hardships. She would sometimes succeed in talking me into accepting the risk. Weeks later, she would invariably let me know that she did overdose after we had talked, but had miraculously survived. She could not resist letting me know how she had swindled me.

Treatment contracts can help avoid such risky and destructive scenarios.

Treatment Contracts

Most important transactions are secured by contracts. Therapy is a long-term working relationship that involves life-and-death risks. A contract can help define each participant's responsibility for managing these risks. It can bring order to a process that may at times feel bewildering.

A treatment contract will help define the limits of what you can expect of your therapist. It also will help define your own responsibility in therapy and fortify your capacity for self-control.

If you are borderline, you are likely to test limits and pounce upon any ambiguity in your treatment agreement. The more details that can be spelled out in writing from the beginning of treatment the better. Developing the contract is the joint responsibility of you and your therapist.

How Well Do Contracts Work?

If you are borderline, you probably have a strong sense of right and wrong. When you give your word, you will do everything in your power to keep it because honor is important to you. That is another consequence of your black-and-white thinking.

You may also have a keen eye for loopholes, so it is important for your contracts to be clear and precise. While you may be given to keeping secrets and committing lies of omission, you are likely to be truthful when questioned directly.

In my experience, well-written contracts are helpful. They are most effective when there is a strong bond between patient and therapist and when their terms are reviewed periodically.

Not only are contracts helpful in outpatient psychotherapy, they can be particularly helpful in defining the ground rules of hospitalization. Hospitalization is a time of emotional crisis that can be particularly treacherous when the expectations of the participants are poorly defined. The next chapter will address some of the pitfalls and opportunities that the hospital presents.

When Sara next sat in my office, she was still livid with anger. She lambasted Jonathan mercilessly. How could she be married to such an ineffectual weakling? He couldn't be trusted to keep her children safe. And he had stood by helplessly all those nights she had been out carousing, never even questioning her whereabouts. If he had been half a man, he would have stopped her before she met with disaster.

Sara then turned her wrath on me. I'd had plenty of time to cure her. Why was she still so sick that she could not even enjoy a vacation at the beach? Why was the dream still haunting her? Why was she so full of fear and hate? She had been crazy to trust me. She would never get well in my hands.

When Sara's tirade ended, I asked her to tell me again what happened at the beach. She recalled watching Jonathan playing with Lisa in the surf, just like her daddy used to play with her. She had suddenly felt panicky as if her children were in danger. That was when she looked for Megan and couldn't find her. All she could think about was saving her baby. As she ran through the water, she momentarily saw not Jonathan, but her daddy lifting the child overhead. And she flashed back to the awful moments that those same strong arms had swept her from her bed deep in the night.

Sara was overcome with anguish by the image of the father she had adored and trusted juxtaposed with the image of the father she dreaded. She could not imagine that the two were the same man. She looked at Jonathan playing so lovingly with her children and wondered how he would eventually betray them.

Now she regarded me, too, with suspicion. She felt much too vulnerable in my care, particularly when she realized that her urgency to return home from the beach was fueled by her yearning for the safety of my presence. She had hoped that I would comfort her and make the pain go away. Instead, I had brought the origin of her pain into sharper focus.

Sara set out over the following weeks to prove she had no need for me. She cancelled the next two appointments, saying she had to stay home with sick children. When I saw her next she had lost weight and was beginning to look emaciated. She brushed off my concern, declaring that it was none of my business how much she weighed. She would diet as long as she pleased until she felt as thin as she needed to be. For now she had no need to eat.

Sara would not acknowledge that her hunger strike was connected in any way with the fast she had undertaken as a teenager. While she was vaguely aware of its meaning as a declaration of independence, she missed entirely the red flag that signalled her enduring feelings of defectiveness and her need to punish herself for some still unnamed sin.

Sara's dwindling size soon took center stage in her treatment. The thinner she got, the more she engaged me in a struggle to interrupt her self-destructive behavior. When I told her that she would be hospitalized if she lost another five pounds, she threatened to leave treatment. But she was already in serious danger. She was malnourished and severely dehydrated.

One hot summer day, while pushing her children on the swings at the park, she passed out. By the time the ambulance reached her, she was barely breathing. And on the way to the hospital emergency room, her heart stopped beating.

13

Hospitalization

"Bred en bawn in a brier-patch, Brer Fox."

"DE TAR BABY"
JOEL CHANDLER HARRIS, 1892

"I just don't see the point," Rose told me on the telephone late on a Friday afternoon.

"What do you mean?" I asked, already knowing what was coming next. We had had similar conversations time and again.

". . . in going on. I don't see the point in going on," Rose replied. "I'm just no use to anyone."

"Are you thinking again about killing yourself?" I asked.

"I'm not saying. I know what you'll do if I tell you. You'll put me in the hospital again." There was a pause. "But I have these pills left over from the other doctor, and I can't help thinking about going to sleep and never having to wake up."

"It certainly sounds like you do need to be in the hospital," I said.

"No, No!" Rose protested. "You know how much I hate it there. Please don't do this to me."

After lengthy debate, Rose finally agreed to be admitted to the hospital. I breathed a sigh of relief. She was a frail and gentle woman in her mid-60s. It made me shudder to think about sending the sheriff's deputies to bring her forcibly to the hospital. There would have been no choice, however, if she did not agree to go.

This scene always came out the same, with Rose saving face for both of us, but each time it carried the same level of suspense. This time, she told me upon her arrival at the hospital that she had impulsively taken "a handful" of pills just before leaving home.

For Rose, the hospital was an intricate briar patch. She truly despised the confinement, the prying eyes and ears of the staff, and the regimented schedule of group therapy and activities. But she felt safe and secure there with nurses always close by. For a little while, she did not have to fight loneliness or boredom or make decisions. And she would usually make one or two new friends who would be her link to the world for the next few weeks or months.

If you are borderline, you will probably spend some time in the hospital on your way to recovery. As in Rose's case, your ticket of admission will most likely be health-threatening or life-threatening behavior. Also like Rose, the hospital will hold for you a mixture of foreboding and allure. Once within its bosom, it may become difficult to venture back outside.

Unless you have the willingness and resources to commit to a long-term inpatient program of a year or more's duration, it is best to measure your hospital stay in days. One way to contain your stay is by making a contract with your doctor that spells out in advance the length of stay and specific goals of treatment.

The principal goal of short-term hospitalization is to restore safety. This is approached initially by containing the dangerous behavior that triggered hospital admission. Besides maintaining safety, prevention of impulsive behavior helps to expose the painful feelings behind it so that these feelings can be discussed. Talking about these underlying emotions is one of the keys to lasting behavior control.

Sometimes the hospital provides enough physical and emotional security to allow new memories and feelings to emerge. We then not only can prevent our fragile ancient vessel from disintegrating, but can perhaps recover a few key fragments that help it to take shape.

Hospitalization also may be an opportunity to restore normal patterns of sleep and healthy eating habits, reevaluate priorities, and reengage in dialogue with key people in your life. In addition to preventing direct physical damage to yourself, it is a means of controlling the damage that may occur in your relationships, your job, and your lifestyle at times of crisis.

A realistic time frame for accomplishing these basic goals is ten to fourteen days. Beyond this looms a serious risk of addiction to the hospital. Despite your best intentions to stay within the contract, you may find yourself looking for ways to prolong your stay. By direct threat or by hint and innuendo, you may let the staff know that you are still in danger and, therefore, cannot be discharged. Unless you can be transferred to a state hospital or other facility that can offer ongoing safety in an alternative place, time limits can always be defeated. The price of these short-term victories, however, is high. The trauma of your eventual departure from the hospital increases with every day you stay.

The longer you remain in the hospital, the more it will become a stage for playing out your inner conflicts. You will choose your champions among the staff and pit them against those you decide are the enemy. You will test the limits of the rules and the staff's capacity to enforce them. You may even test the physical limits of the hospital by fleeing from it, at the same time testing the staff's ability and willingness to protect you.

Once a power struggle develops, you may lose sight of your

reasons for coming to the hospital and of your treatment goals. You may also devalue your doctor's and the hospital's capacity to help you. The flaws you detect in the treatment team may justify your rejection of it and cause you to disengage from treatment. Keep in mind that black-and-white thinking, unforgiving of flaws, is central to what keeps you at odds with others and with yourself.

Maintaining perspective is crucial to the effective use of your time in the hospital. You have a right to complain about the housekeeping, the food, or a late medication. You owe it to yourself, however, not to let such issues take over the time you need in therapy to devote to more personal matters.

Your relationship with your doctor and the treatment staff is a partnership to promote your health. Treatment will progress if all members of the team keep the specific goals of your stay firmly in mind and respect the need to keep it short.

Meg was a thirty-eight-year-old sales representative who was admitted to the hospital because of a suicide attempt in the midst of a marital crisis. Several days into her stay, she became sexually involved with a twenty-year-old college student who had been admitted because of delusions of grandeur.

Meg let her social worker and selected nurses know about her liaison with the young man, but kept it scrupulously hidden from the other patients, who were aware only of an apparently innocent friendship between the two.

Because a sexual affair was not only against hospital rules, but also risked undermining both patients' treatments, the staff felt obligated to limit the contact between them. They were no longer permitted to be alone together on the unit and were locked out of their bedrooms during the day.

Meg artfully used these measures to pit the patient group against the authority of the staff. She accused the staff of having dirty minds for obstructing a friendship that was providing mutual emotional support. The restrictions seemed outrageous to the other patients in the face of her scenario. She succeeded in engendering mistrust among the entire group.

Meg knew the rules of treatment well. She relied on the staff's obligation to maintain confidentiality in order to keep the contest for her peers' loyalty unbalanced. She even challenged my willingness to respect her confidentiality by attacking me verbally over this issue during group therapy. After I sustained her attack without counterattacking or breaking her trust, she began to engage in treatment.

Hospital treatment provides an opportunity to integrate a variety of treatment modalities. In the safety of the hospital, medications can often be regulated more quickly than at home. Individual therapy may occur daily in order to work intensively on a specific problem. Family therapy may help resolve impasses in your relationships and define the roles of your significant others in your treatment. Finally, group therapy offers a unique opportunity to compare experiences with others and to receive feedback from peers about your perceptions and behavior. The next chapter will explore the special role of group therapy in treating BPD.

My next meeting with Sara was in a hospital room reminiscent of our first encounter. Instead of the vibrant and engaging woman I first met, however, this time I found her frail and haggard. She was dressed in a plain hospital gown, her hair pulled back to make way for an oxygen mask that covered her nose and mouth. An intravenous line was in place just beneath her collarbone. A clear plastic feeding tube dangled from her nose beneath the mask. She could barely speak.

"How could you let this happen to me?" Sara's first words tore at my heart with an accusation that echoed my own thoughts. I had miscalculated the margin of safety. If not for the prompt response of the rescue team and the efforts of the emergency room crisis team, Sara would have died.

Over the next several days as she regained her strength, Sara took every opportunity to remind me how I had let her down. She used her helpless and pitiful appearance, encumbered with tubes and monitors, to twist the knife deeper. She played on my guilt to try to enlist me as an ally in her efforts to undermine the medical team's work to restore her to health. She complained bitterly of the nasogastric tube that was bringing her body the nourishment she had so stubbornly shunned. She begged to have it removed.

I resisted the temptation to indulge her plea for rescue and worked with the medical team to establish realistic goals for the acute phase of her recovery. We agreed that she would have to gain at least ten pounds before she could be taken off bedrest and fifteen pounds before the feeding tube could be safely removed. Her internist and I together discussed these criteria with Sara in order to emphasize our agreement about them. Sara was told that she could eat, even with the feeding tube in place. She could therefore influence how quickly these goals were reached.

Once the rules had been clearly defined, Sara relaxed and began to eat. Since she was no longer in control of what went into her body, she was no longer responsible for it either and needed no longer to punish herself. Besides, her brush with death and the treatment itself were punishment enough. She quickly met the medical goals and was transferred to the psychiatric unit. There we followed up promptly with a treatment contract in which various levels of freedom and choice depended on stages of weight gain and her cooperation with the treatment program.

Sara vocally protested her hospital confinement. She argued with most of the staff when it was time for her to attend group therapy or other activities. She begged for extra privileges and became irate when they turned her down. Only one nurse, an energetic woman in her early thirties, escaped her wrath. She was firm and direct with Sara from the start, and Sara quickly stopped testing her limits. When Betty was on duty, Sara felt secure and softened her hostile stance.

I remained the target of Sara's most intense rage. She treated me, from the start, like a jailer. The time to have hospitalized her, she contended, was before her collapse. Now that she was better, it was no longer necessary. She accused me of keeping her in the hospital so that I could hide behind the staff because I was afraid to deal with her anger by myself. Her radar for my self-doubts was uncanny, and I began to wonder whether she was right. But I also wondered what we were reenacting from Sara's past.

"This wasn't the first time someone failed to keep you safe," I remarked during one of Sara's tirades. Sara fell silent. Her eyes filled with tears. As she sobbed, her mind filled with a thought that she had banished years ago.

"Why didn't she take me away from him?" She could feel the contempt rising within her. "If she really loved me, why did she let it keep happening?"

Sara had identified another villain in the piece. Her mother was an accomplice to her father's brutality because of her failure to leave or stand up to him. She had been a weakling, like the nurses Sara despised for not standing up to her. If only she had been strong like Betty.

"She got what she deserved," Sara remarked. The words were familiar and we both recalled Sara's comment following her own brutal beating at the hands of a stranger. She was flooded with guilt when she realized that she had had the same thought as a child while her mother lay battered on the floor one too many times.

14

Group Therapy

It takes one to know one.

ANONYMOUS SEVEN-YEAR-OLD

It is often easier to recognize problems in others than to see the same problems in ourselves. If you are borderline, you are probably expert at picking out borderline behaviors in others.

In 1989, as part of the same burst of honesty that spawned this book, we started a borderline behaviors group on the inpatient unit that I directed. We began by providing handouts on BPD and explaining to the participants why they had been included in the group. For many, this first group was therapeutic. They expressed relief and gratitude to have both a name for their suffering that made sense to them and a clear framework for developing goals.

Soon after the group began, something marvelous began to happen. Within hours of new admissions to the unit, the veterans in the group would approach the group leader and say, "You know, Julie really needs to be in your group." Invariably, they would be right.

Their intuitive diagnosis foresaw the outcome of the formal evaluation that followed.

That same perceptiveness lay at the heart of the group process. As members discussed their emotional and interpersonal struggles, their peers identified their borderline behaviors and the distorted perceptions that lay behind them. Having identified these behaviors in those around them, each member became increasingly aware of similar behaviors in herself. The group members in this way served as mirrors for each other to see themselves more clearly.

The group members brimmed with energy and enthusiasm and carried their confrontations with each other beyond the confines of the group. The group leader and the structure of the group helped to keep these confrontations appropriate and to contain any aggressive component of their spirited competitiveness. The bonds among the group members were primarily supportive and caring. Even conflicts arising outside the group could often be resolved within the group by identifying how each antagonist's borderline thinking contributed to the fight.

The group fast became a favorite activity among its participants, who often identified it as the richest learning experience of their stay. As a result, an outpatient group was formed so that the learning could continue beyond the brief time frame of the hospital stay.

As with individual therapy, the therapy group should have a contract that clearly spells out rules of conduct. Confidentiality is of paramount importance. Clear communication, owning one's own feelings and behavior, and mutual respect should be addressed.

A basic principle of most outpatient therapy groups is that socialization outside the group is forbidden. There is a great temptation, particularly among lonely and anxious participants, to seek solace in each other's company. This can seriously undermine the group's trust and safety. Factions may form that exclude some members. Confidentiality is at greater risk when members meet socially.

Most importantly, the emotional safety of the group is founded upon the members' anonymity and neutrality toward one another. Risking exposure of embarrassing secrets becomes much harder if the emotional investment in other members reaches beyond the group's boundaries.

A strong and knowledgeable leader is essential to maintaining the group rules and keeping it on track. Leading such a group is for neither the inexperienced nor the faint of heart. The leader's own boundaries must stand up to the emotional storm that the group can generate. A cotherapist can help the group stay focused.

Group therapy is not a substitute for individual therapy. All patients in borderline groups should also be required to have an individual therapist. Free exchange of information between therapists is important if they are to work together on your behalf. The individual therapist retains primary responsibility for intervening at times of crisis, with interventions guided by the individual treatment contract.

Leaving victimhood behind is a central goal of treatment. If you are borderline, you have lived life so far seemingly at the mercy of others, of fate, and of your own impulses. Group therapy is designed for change. It is an opportunity to learn new ways to make decisions, communicate effectively, and manage your relationships. It is a chance for members to try on new behaviors and model their effectiveness for each other. Group therapy is the privilege of tapping the collective problem-solving capability of an unusually creative and resourceful group of people.

Just as BPD develops out of an interplay of biological and environmental factors, so treatment enlists both biological and psychological interventions. If individual and group therapy help to gather the fragments up and fit them together, therapeutic drugs are often part of the glue that holds them together. The next chapter will examine the use of medications in the treatment of BPD.

*S*ara's rage gave way to profound sadness when she realized how truly defenseless she had been. She had always believed that her mother had cared for her and kept her safe despite the horrible scenes with her drunken father. Now she felt completely abandoned.

One night Sara dreamed that she had died. As she looked down upon her own grave, a child approached, a boy of fourteen. He stood before the grave and wept. She did not recognize him, but he seemed familiar. She felt sorry for his grief and wanted to comfort him, but he could not see her. Then the scene changed and she watched him running frantically through the woods, lost and frightened. She awakened drenched in sweat.

When Sara told me the dream for the first time, I asked her to close her eyes and describe it again as if it were happening right then, but to imagine it through the child's eyes. When she found herself in front of the grave, I asked her to read the inscription on the headstone. There beneath her own maiden name she read, "born May 17, 1956, died February 23, 1976."

Sara opened her eyes in bewilderment. I reminded her that she had dreamed many times about a lost child. Then she understood. She was not the only child that had been abandoned by a derelict mother. In the depths of her soul, she had kept the memory of a child that would have been, had she not ended her pregnancy out of desperate fear of her father's anger. In her imagination, she had aged him as time passed until he appeared to her in her dream at age fourteen.

Sara wailed with grief. The rage that had permeated our relationship for so many weeks was for all the parents who had failed to protect their children. If Sara was to continue to heal, she would need to find a way to forgive us all.

I marveled at the richness of meaning in Sara's dream as it gave up its secrets and provided a window to her heart. Dreams represent ideas by symbols and often condense many ideas within *a single succinct image. The dates on the gravestone meant that life as she had known it ended for Sara on the day of the abortion. On that day something essential within her had died. It marked the death of her close and loving relationship with her father. And of course the dream also referred to the literal death of the child that might have been. The figure gazing at the grave was also its legitimate occupant. One mystery remained. Why had Sara always imagined that the child would have been a boy?*

As Sara regained her stamina, she began attending the inpatient therapy group where another drama unfolded. Sara had entered the group tentatively, refusing at first to speak. But as she began to share with the group some of her new discoveries about herself, she soon moved to center stage. Her need for attention in the group may have resulted in part from my being the group leader. For many days she undermined all my efforts to include others in the process. She pouted visibly whenever my attention was focused on someone else.

When one day a young man in his mid-twenties joined the group, Sara's attitude suddenly changed. She not only gave up her place in the spotlight, but took every opportunity to direct my attention and the group's to this man. He was, on the surface, hateful and calloused, unappealing to most of the group. But Sara's determination to help him was relentless.

Tom was a handsome man despite the many scars on his face and body that chronicled a life of brawling and living on the brink. With his square jaw and slightly hooked nose, he strongly resembled Dick Tracy. The resemblance stopped, however, at his sandy blond hair that fell almost randomly from the part in the middle to his shoulders.

Tom had been admitted because of episodes of explosive rage that had caused his wife of two years to leave him. She had felt so threatened that she had obtained a restraining order to prevent him from coming near her after they separated. She was still in love with him, however, and had promised to consider a reconciliation if he got treatment and changed his ways.

Sara had been drawn to Tom from the start. He was mysterious and colorful like the men who had attracted her before she met Jonathan. But her attraction to this man was neither sexual nor romantic. What drew her to him was something inexplicably tragic beneath his hardened demeanor. She was determined to learn the secrets of his past.

In the eyes of others, Sara and Tom were becoming involved romantically. They were virtually inseparable in the hospital and sat next to each other in every group. Since Sara's male friends had always been lovers in the past, her behavior toward him was somewhat provocative. Their relationship caused a stir among the staff, who were troubled by their infringement upon the rules regarding the boundaries of physical contact in the hospital, and among the patients, who saw their relationship as setting them apart from the rest of the patient group. Since they were both married, the forbidden quality of their apparent liaison was also titillating.

The reaction of others to their relationship provided a powerful distraction from the painful business of therapy. Sara and Tom became deeply invested in defending their honor and their right to be friends. I, too, was distracted by the pressure from the staff for me, as Sara's doctor, to get her to behave herself.

It is a remarkable irony that the very symptoms and behaviors that arise in order to keep painful memories and feelings hidden are also symbolic clues to the content of these experiences. So our mutual engagement in the struggle over Sara's involvement with Tom kept us from understanding that it represented something crucial from Sara's past.

15

Drug Therapy

The Lord lets the herbs grow out of the soil
And a wise person does not scorn them.

SIRACH 38:4
THE APOCRYPHA

There is no drug specifically for BPD. Drugs may sometimes be helpful for treating specific symptoms of BPD or to address other illnesses that may occur during the course of BPD. Drugs can help to regulate mood, to reduce anxiety, to control impulses—including the urge to self-mutilate—to reduce the frequency of dissociative symptoms, and to correct misperceptions of reality such as hallucinations or feelings of persecution.

This chapter will identify the most commonly used types of medications and why they are usually prescribed. It will identify significant advantages and disadvantages of each drug type. Drugs within each category will be listed by their generic name. Their most common trade names will be found in parentheses.

While this chapter has been updated for the millennium, drug therapy is a dynamically changing field. Both new drugs and new applications for existing drugs regularly become available.

Antidepressants

Depression, lasting from hours to months, occurs commonly with BPD. Depression affects mood, thinking, activity level, and biological functions such as sleep, appetite, energy level, and sexual drive. Typical thought patterns in depression include feelings of helplessness, hopelessness, worthlessness, and guilt. Thoughts and activity may be painfully slow or sometimes frenzied. The most typical biological changes include frequent awakenings during the night, early-morning awakening, loss of appetite and weight, and loss of energy. The middle- and early-morning awakening pattern of insomnia strongly suggests depression and indicates the likelihood of response to antidepressant medications.

Antidepressants should be considered when biological symptoms are prominent and have been present for more than a week or two. The presence of suicidal thoughts would be another reason to consider using antidepressants early in treatment. Antidepressants are sometimes also used, however, to modify the painful feelings, or dysphoria, that frequently arise in BPD. They may also help curb many of the impulsive behaviors associated with BPD.

The older generation of antidepressants, or tricyclic antidepressants (TCAs), treated depression as effectively as the newer drugs commonly used today. The most widely used TCAs were amitriptyline (Elavil), nortriptyline (Pamelor), imipramine (Tofranil), desipramine (Norpramin), and doxepin (Sinequan). Their most important drawback was that they are all potentially lethal in overdose. Given the frequency of suicidal behavior in people with BPD, this risk is significant. Even at therapeutic doses, TCAs can cause rhythm disturbances of the heart in certain susceptible people. They also have a number of uncomfortable side effects, including particularly drowsiness, dizziness, dry mouth, constipation, and blurred near vision.

While TCAs are not generally the first antidepressant choice today, they are still in use. Some people, for unknown reasons, respond better to a TCA than to any of the newer drugs. TCAs are also considerably less expensive than the newer drugs because they are all available generically. Sometimes, small doses of sedating TCAs, such as amitriptyline or doxepin, or trazodone (Desyrel), a closely related drug with properties similar to TCAs, are used to treat insomnia. They often maintain their effectiveness longer than conventional sedatives and are less prone to developing addiction.

If you are prescribed a TCA, your doctor may prescribe it in limited quantities to limit your risk of overdosing with it. It is important for you to take it as prescribed. If you change medications or have extra medication left over for any reason, you should turn it in to your doctor or dispose of it. While this is especially important for TCAs, it is a good rule for dealing with all medications. Stockpiling medications can offer dangerous temptations at times of emotional pain.

The selective serotonin reuptake inhibitor (SSRI) antidepressants were the first of a new generation of antidepressants that offer a safer alternative to the tricyclic antidepressants. While overdoses may still be fatal, survival is far more likely with an overdose of an SSRI than with a TCA. These medications, which now include fluoxetine (Prozac), sertraline (Zoloft), paroxetine (Paxil), fluvoxamine (Luvox), and citalopram (Celexa), have become powerful tools in treating depression and various forms of anxiety. Because the SSRIs are generally free of the sedation and mental clouding that is common with the TCAs, people often feel more normal on the newer drugs. No drug is entirely free of side effects, however. For the SSRIs, perhaps the most vexing of side effects has been sexual dysfunction, including problems with both arousal and reaching orgasm.

SSRIs have been helpful in limiting the depths of despair that many people with BPD experience as well as controlling panic attacks and other overwhelming feelings that often lead to self-destructive behaviors. For some people, these drugs significantly reduce the urge to self-mutilate or to engage in other mood-altering behaviors such as bingeing and purging.

Since the SSRIs have been available, they have been found to be helpful in treating an expanding number of conditions and symptoms, many of which may coexist with BPD. They have been particularly effective in treating Panic Disorder and Obsessive-Compulsive Disorder. They have also been helpful in preventing premenstrual mood changes, controlling the bingeing and purging of bulimia, reducing the discomfort of fibromyalgia, and decreasing the self-consciousness and shyness of Social Phobia.

Other new-generation antidepressants include nefazadone (Serzone), venlafaxine (Effexor), bupropion (Wellbutrin), and mirtazapine (Remeron). These drugs share the safety profile of the SSRIs and their potency in treating depression, but may not share their broad efficacy in treating other disorders. They may, however, offer other advantages. Nefazodone is less likely to cause sexual dysfunction than the SSRIs while still sharing many of their characteristics. Both bupropion and mirtazapine not only are free of sexual dysfunction, but each can sometimes restore normal sexual function when added to an SSRI. They may also enhance the antidepressant effect of the SSRIs when used in combination. Their side-effect profiles are very different from one another in other respects, however. Bupropion is stimulating and not at all sedating and seldom causes weight gain. Mirtazapine is very sedating, an advantage if insomnia has been severe, but sometimes difficult to tolerate early in treatment. Mirtazapine frequently causes weight gain, its most troubling side effect. Venlafaxine has been found in some studies to be helpful for some people who have responded poorly to a variety of other agents.

By the time this book is in print, reboxetine (Vestra), which belongs to a new class of antidepressants known as selective nor-epinephrine reuptake inhibitors, will likely be available. Claims from pre-marketing trials include efficacy at least equivalent to the TCAs and SSRIs, a more rapid onset of action, and a relatively benign side-effect profile. Such claims must now, however, survive the test of time when used in much larger numbers of patients.

Monoamine oxidase inhibitors, including phenelzine (Nardil) and tranylcypromine (Parnate), are a lesser used but highly effective class of antidepressants. These may be particularly effective if you have atypical biological symptoms (e.g., sleeping too much, increased appetite, weight gain), phobias, preoccupation with physical symptoms, or depressions that are triggered by rejection. They are sometimes effective when more conventional agents have failed.

Unfortunately, the MAOIs can have serious interactions with certain other drugs and even common foods, such as aged wine and cheese, that can cause life-threatening elevations of blood pressure or muscle rigidity and mental confusion. Because of these risks, they are used infrequently. For some people, however, if the food and drug restrictions are scrupulously followed, MAOIs can have potent mood-stabilizing and anxiety-relieving effects.

If you are prescribed an antidepressant medication, you will need to be patient, something not so easy for people with BPD, in awaiting its effects. Antidepressants must be taken on a regularly scheduled basis in order to be effective. It typically takes two to four weeks for the antidepressant effects to develop. As a rule, side effects occur early and fade with time, while therapeutic effects occur later and increase with time. Occasionally improvement can be seen within days, but this is an exception to the rule.

While the effects of antidepressants can be worth waiting for, they are not a panacea for the mood disturbances that occur in BPD. They can be very helpful when depressed mood has been sustained over weeks and months, particularly when it has been accompanied by disturbances in sleep, appetite, and energy level. They may not, however, prevent the emotional crashes that can occur in the face of a broken relationship or other perceived abandonment or failure.

Many patients will respond equally well to any of the newer antidepressants, but some will do better on a specific drug. Finding the best match of medication to patient then becomes a matter of trial and error that often requires patience and persistence. Because antidepressants may take weeks to relieve symptoms, it is crucial not to abandon any medication too hastily.

Mood-Stabilizing Agents

Mood-stabilizing drugs have been studied primarily in the treatment of patients with Bipolar Disorder (once known as Manic-Depressive Disorder), but are increasingly being used by some clinicians to treat the drastic mood changes that can also occur in BPD. In addition to their mood-stabilizing effects, these agents can also be helpful in modifying explosive rage and aggression, both when directed at others and when directed at the self in the form of self-mutilation. This can be invaluable if explosive outbursts threaten to destroy valued relationships before psychotherapy can be completed.

When depressed moods are accompanied by rage, mood stabilizers may be a safer alternative to antidepressants, since the latter may sometimes worsen irritability and aggressiveness, particularly early in treatment. These drugs are often combined with the antidepressants and may enhance their effects when the response to treatment has been incomplete.

Lithium (Lithonate, Eskalith, Lithobid), the oldest known mood-stabilizing drug, has been widely used since the 1960s. Lithium produces few uncomfortable side effects at therapeutic doses, but poses significant risk and may even be lethal if the blood level gets too high. Many things, including particularly dehydration and interactions with other drugs, can push lithium blood levels outside of the drug's narrow therapeutic range and pose danger. Lithium can also affect thyroid, kidney, and cardiac function. Periodic monitoring with blood tests is required to maintain an appropriate level and detect adverse effects.

Several agents originally developed to treat seizures have been found to have powerful mood-stabilizing effects. Valproate (Depakote) is the antiseizure medication most commonly used by psychiatrists today to control mood swings. It has been generally well-tolerated but can sometimes affect liver function and must be monitored periodically with blood tests. Carbamazepine (Tegretol) is an older drug that has also been used widely as a mood stabilizer. It carries a risk, however, of drastically reducing the number of infection-fighting white blood cells and must also be monitored closely. It's a rare complication, but it can be life-threatening.

Data is accumulating on a rapidly growing list of related agents, including gabapentin (Neurontin), lamotrigine (Lamictal), and topiramate (Topamax), among others. As with the antidepressants, these drugs are generally selected for each patient according to the drug's side effects and risks as much as for differences in their clinical effects. All of the antiseizure drugs are helpful in relieving certain kinds of chronic pain. Gabapentin appears also to have anxiety-relieving effects. Lamotrigine may be most effective in restoring normal mood in depressed patients but can occasionally cause very severe rashes and liver damage. Topiramate is unique among these agents in its tendency to cause weight loss rather than weight gain.

Major Tranquilizers

The major tranquilizers, or antipsychotic drugs, have long been used to treat some of the symptoms of BPD. They can be most helpful in treating dissociative symptoms and in controlling self-destructive impulses. They may be the most effective treatment for the intense anxiety that often occurs in BPD. They can also reduce or eliminate hallucinations or paranoid thoughts. Some of their effects, such as curbing the impulse to self-mutilate, may be seen with as little as a single dose, while others may require regular dosing over weeks or months.

Major tranquilizers are not addictive. Their most significant drawback is a group of side effects that include various involuntary movements. Of most concern is tardive dyskinesia, a movement disorder usually beginning with involuntary movements of the mouth and tongue that is often permanent, even after drugs are withdrawn. While this usually occurs after long exposure to high doses, it can occasionally arise early in treatment. The risk can be minimized with careful monitoring for appearance of the earliest signs. When used appropriately, major tranquilizers can be a life-saving intervention with benefits that far outweigh the risks.

Tardive dyskinesia and other movement disorders occur most commonly with the older drugs, such as haloperidol (Haldol), thiothixene (Navane), trifluoperazine (Stelazine), thioridazine (Mellaril), and chlorpromazine (Thorazine). As with the antidepressants, a new generation of major tranquilizers has emerged that has fewer uncomfortable side effects than the older drugs. Clozapine (Clozaril), the first of the newer drugs, appears particularly free of involuntary movements and the risk of tardive dyskinesia. Good things, however, often come at a price. Clozapine produces a small but significant incidence of agranulocytosis, a loss of infection-fighting white blood cells that can be fatal. The drug can only be administered when monitored closely with weekly blood tests.

Other new-generation major tranquilizers include risperidone (Risperdal), olanzapine (Zyprexa), and quetiapine (Seroquel). While experience with using these drugs on a long-term basis is still very limited, a significantly reduced risk of tardive dyskinesia also looks promising. By the time you read this, additional entries to the field may be available that have been developed to duplicate the advantages of these newer drugs with even fewer risks. As with the antidepressants, some people may still respond better to the older drugs, which are also considerably less expensive than the newer ones. The older drugs may be used with relative safety when administered for short periods of time or used only occasionally.

Minor Tranquilizers

Minor tranquilizers, or benzodiazepines, are commonly prescribed to control anxiety and to promote sleep. They work quickly on a dose-for-dose basis and wear off between doses. They cause drowsiness and, like alcohol, can increase the risk of traffic accidents, especially if taken just before driving. While they are relatively free of uncomfortable side effects or toxicity, they present special hazards if you are borderline and thus should be used with caution.

Minor tranquilizers are both physically and psychologically addictive. Physical addiction means that after taking them regularly for weeks or months, you may have potentially dangerous withdrawal symptoms if you stop taking them abruptly. Psychological addiction means that you may have difficulty stopping them because their effects are immediate, dramatic, and pleasurable. Once you have experienced these effects, you may not be able to resist repeating the experience. Minor tranquilizers often lose their effectiveness with time, resulting in gradually increasing doses. Escalation of the dose, in turn, increases the risk of addiction. Keeping the dose low and duration of use brief can help limit the risk of addiction.

While minor tranquilizers are usually calming, they can make some people irritable or even aggressive. Like alcohol, minor tranquilizers can impair self-control, leading to impulsive behavior and poor judgment. They can trigger flashbacks and other dissociative symptoms and can worsen depression over time. They therefore have a limited role in treating BPD and, when used, should be closely monitored.

Longer-acting drugs, such as clonazepam (Klonopin) and chlorazepate (Tranxene), may be slightly safer than shorter-acting drugs, such as lorazepam (Ativan), alprazolam (Xanax), and triazolam (Halcion). They may be less prone to withdrawal symptoms because they leave the body slowly even when stopped abruptly. They may be less psychologically addictive because their effects are more gradual and subtle. They may also be less apt to cause lapses of memory or to trigger dissociative events.

Alprazolam has been approved for use in treating panic attacks. In the dose range recommended for preventing panic attacks, the likelihood of eventual addiction is high and may be overwhelming if you are borderline. Safer alternatives, such as the SSRI antidepressants, are available and highly effective.

Two new drugs for sleep, zolpidem (Ambien) and zaleplon (Sonata), represent a separate class of sedatives distinct from the benzodiazepines. They have been claimed to be relatively free both of addiction potential and the need for dose escalation over time. The jury is still out on both counts. What is clearly special about these drugs, however, is that they are so short-acting that they rarely leave a hangover. In fact, they can even be taken in the middle of a sleepless night without interfering with the next morning's alertness. Like the benzodiazepines, their use should be time-limited and closely monitored.

Buspirone (BuSpar) is a unique, non-benzodiazepine antianxiety agent that is not addicting and, for the most part, non-sedating. Buspirone is often combined with an SSRI antidepressant. When so combined, buspirone may enhance the antidepressant and antianxiety effects of the SSRI. For some people, it may also counteract the sexual side effects of the SSRIs. Like antidepressants, buspirone must be taken regularly over a period of weeks in order to realize its full anxiety-relieving effects.

Anxiety and insomnia are best treated without drugs whenever possible. Avoiding alcohol and caffeine, exercising regularly, and learning how to manage specific stressful situations may go a long way toward helping you relax. Relaxation techniques and meditation are easily learned ways to relieve tension. Providing soothing surroundings with calming colors, tranquil music, and physical comfort can help.

Narcotic Antagonists

One other drug that merits mention is naltrexone (ReVia). This drug, which blocks the effects of narcotics on the nervous system, was originally studied as a treatment for narcotics addiction. More recently, it has been found also to limit the craving for alcohol in some alcoholics. Naltrexone may also reduce the urge to self-mutilate in patients with a variety of diagnoses. While it is not clear how helpful this drug will turn out to be in preventing self-mutilation in BPD, it is worth watching. It may even be worth trying for some people who struggle both with chemical addictions and compulsive self-injury.

Combining Medications

When treating BPD, experienced clinicians often blend medications from the various classes described above. Sometimes, they may even prescribe more than one medication of the same type. Possible drug interactions must be considered, not only among these medications, but also between these medications and those that are prescribed for other medical problems. There may even be interactions between prescription medications and herbal remedies or nutritional supplements. It is important to tell any physician who is prescribing for you about all medications, herbs, and supplements you may be taking. Even some foods, such as grapefruit juice, can significantly affect the blood levels and actions of certain drugs.

Using Medicines Wisely

If your doctor recommends that you take medication, find out all that you need to know to take it properly. Ask whether the drug is to be taken regularly, as is usually the case with antidepressants and mood-stabilizing medications, or only when you have symptoms. Ask whether there are dangerous side effects and what reasons might arise to prompt you to stop taking the drug.

Make sure that your doctor knows about every other medication you are taking, including birth control pills and nonprescription remedies. Take herbal remedies or supplements only with your doctor's knowledge and approval. If there is any doubt, bring a list of ingredients for your doctor to see. Treatment failures or adverse reactions with therapeutic drugs can often be traced to the effects of other substances, such as herbal stimulants in diet preparations, that patients had not thought important enough to mention or had not wanted to give up.

Prescribing medication is an act of trust between you and your doctor. Let your doctor know if you are uncomfortable in any way about taking medication or if you develop side effects. Maintain your end of the trust by using medication to reach the goals that you are working toward together and by not damaging yourself or your treatment relationship.

*A*clue to Tom's significance for Sara came one day during group therapy when Tom attacked me verbally. He had had numerous arguments with the nurses about his flagrant disregard for hospital rules and had begun to feel singled out for punishment. He had decided that the real issue was his relationship with Sara and had assumed that I put the nurses up to harassing him so that he would leave my patient alone.

"You're just like my old man," Tom shouted. "You only listen to one side." As Tom warmed to his theme he rose from his chair and took a step toward me. A look of horror crossed Sara's face. She sat transfixed. When I asked Tom to tell us how else his father made him angry, he sat down and began talking about his childhood. There unfolded a tale of terrifying physical abuse at the hands of a drunken father. Sobbing, he recalled how his mother had comforted him after the beatings that she had been helpless to prevent.

When Sara and I next met for individual therapy, she recalled her terror upon thinking that Tom was going to hurt me. Then she described the many similar confrontations that she had witnessed between her brother Mark and her father before Mark left home. Once they had actually exchanged blows, and Sara had feared that Mark would kill him. It was over these fights that the rift between Mark and Sara had formed. She had never understood why Mark so despised her father.

Now the resemblance between Tom and Mark was obvious. Sara and I both guessed that this was the basis for her fascination with Tom. But why would she be so drawn to a man who reminded her of the brother she hated?

Sara's flashbacks resumed with a vengeance. The feeling of the gun barrel against her temple recurred so often and so vividly that she began to feel pain in her temple. The sounds of her father's slaps and her mother's cries were so intense that Sara would cover her ears with her hands, trying vainly to shut them out. She developed severe insomnia, lying awake much of the night with flashbacks and awakening finally around four in the morning. She once again stopped eating, this time not willfully, but because the thought of food nauseated her.

We decided then that the emotional pain had become too intense to bear and that medication was indicated. We had avoided medicating Sara when she was first admitted because of her fragile physical state. Now there was an opportunity to start medication before she had a chance to become malnourished again. An anti-depressant was likely to ease the pain, allow her to sleep, and encourage the return of her appetite. It might also cause the flashbacks to subside. I selected one of the SSRIs because of the relatively rapid action of this class. If her sleep disturbance per-sisted, we could later add a small dose of a more sedating anti-depressant. We continued to avoid using any of the minor tranquilizers both because of Sara's problems with addictions and because these agents sometimes worsened flashbacks.

The flashbacks did subside and Sara began to eat and to sleep. Within two weeks she improved enough to be discharged from the hospital. Sara and her family were grateful to be reunited. She was somewhat apprehensive, however, about leaving the safety of the hospital and the security of daily psychotherapy sessions. We scheduled her first followup appointment for three days after her hospital discharge.

On her second night home, Sara's nightmare came back for the first time in months. This time she began the dream as the child and ended it as the rescuer. From the rescuer's viewpoint she saw that the child was once again a little boy. But this time she recognized him. It was Mark.

16

Healing
Controlling Impulses

Self-reverence, self-knowledge, self-control,
These three alone lead life to sovereign power.
"Oenone"
Alfred, Lord Tennyson

If you have impulsive behavior patterns, they are likely to persist well into therapy and may even emerge powerfully at critical phases of treatment. These behaviors are often dangerous, even life threatening, and at best, impair your capacity to think, learn, and solve problems.

While specific treatment approaches have been designed to treat some of these behaviors, treatment of a single behavior may shift the impulsivity to another area. The problem, after all, is the painful emotions that are common to all these behaviors and the self-destructiveness that follows. The following are some strategies that can help you regain control.

Keep Your Body Healthy
If you are hungry, tired, or run down, your thinking may be clouded and impaired. Getting adequate rest

may go a long way toward putting you back in control. Do not make decisions when you are physically or mentally exhausted. Find out how much sleep you need to stay alert and make getting it a priority.

Eating on a regular schedule, including at least three meals a day, will help provide adequate nutrition, maintain your energy level, and promote alertness and clear thinking. Satisfying your physical hunger may help avert feelings of emptiness and frustration. Moreover, avoiding starvation will help prevent the rebound impulse to binge and promote more consistent and reliable weight control.

You may find that certain foods make you particularly prone to emotional tension. Commonly, foods containing caffeine, theobromine (tea, chocolate), and concentrated simple sugars are the worst offenders, particularly during the premenstrual period. Reducing or eliminating their consumption may significantly reduce emotional tension and self-destructiveness.

Exercise promotes emotional well-being and mental alertness and helps prepare the body for restful nighttime sleep. Vigorous exercise may also help work off some of the negative energy that accompanies feelings of frustration and rage, enabling you to work through these feelings more effectively.

Your exercise should be chosen to provide you with enjoyment and recreation, not just another source of punishment and frustration. It should be something you look forward to. You might also consider this an opportunity for healthy, nonthreatening companionship; for some, however, the peaceful solitude of a good run or workout can be renewing.

Free Your Brain of Chemical Poisons

You need all the brainpower you can muster to manage your emotions and impulses. Alcohol and drugs in any quantity rob you of your reserve. If you are borderline, even minute quantities of alcohol may impair your capacity to inhibit self-destructive impulses, or may trigger dissociation. Abstinence may be your only means of controlling your use of addictive substances. Alcohol and other drugs affect memory and learning, and can make therapy impossible.

Identifying and treating drug dependencies (including prescription tranquilizers and pain medications) is therefore the earliest priority and must pave the way for solving other problems. But even in the absence of drug abuse, abstinence is strongly recommended.

Become Aware of What Makes You Vulnerable

Hunger, exhaustion, and chemical impairment are only a few of the conditions that predispose to acting on impulse. Menstrual cycles, seasons, and other rhythmic changes may be important. You may be particularly vulnerable to certain changes or to the presence or absence of certain people. Even your schedule of therapy sessions may trigger powerful emotional responses.

Keep a diary. Track your mood several times each day at regular intervals. Record any impulsive behavior as soon as possible after it occurs and reconstruct the events leading up to it. Try to record this information as soon as you become aware of the urge and even before you act. Self-awareness is a powerful tool for self-control.

Control Your Surroundings

You move daily through a tangle of sights, sounds, and ideas that influence your emotions. Some of this you control. You choose what music you listen to, what movies you see, what you watch on television, and to some extent, with whom you interact.

Music can powerfully affect emotions. Rhythms and melodies can stir or soothe. Lyrics can directly provoke self-destructive impulses with violent imagery or can stir painful feelings by reminders of past hurts. Becoming aware of how different kinds of music make you feel and act can help you make it a useful tool rather than a destructive force.

Violence and graphic sexual images in the media can also stir powerful feelings, especially when they connect with traumatic past experiences. If you have been raped or molested, for example, watching movies with these themes should be undertaken only after thorough discussion with your therapist. There may be times when these movies would have therapeutic value, particularly if the issues are dealt with sensitively. You should not, however, decide this on your own.

Be Forgiving

Remember that you are starting on a journey. You cannot expect to have perfect control at the beginning. Feeling guilt over your slipups is part of the cycle that keeps compulsions going. If you slip, record it in your diary and let it go emotionally. Turn your energy toward managing any consequences of the slip. For example, return what can be returned from a recent spending spree, and work on budgeting your resources. If you have binged on food, return immediately to regularly scheduled meals and avoid trying to make up for the binge by skipping meals. Be aware that you are doing your best with the tools you have now.

Join a Support Group

These days, there is an "Anonymous" group for almost every conceivable problem or compulsion. These groups provide a nonjudgmental atmosphere for exploring your problems with fellow sufferers.

Many of these groups use the twelve-step recovery model originally developed by Alcoholics Anonymous. This model includes rigorous self-examination and development of scrupulous honesty with yourself and others. It also provides for investment of faith in a higher power that may be conceived in keeping with your individual beliefs.

Support groups offer personal support. Many provide sponsors or other individuals that you can call if you feel vulnerable or tempted to act impulsively. They offer company when loneliness becomes unbearable.

If you are borderline, support groups are not a substitute for treatment. They are a helpful adjunct that can provide safety, security, and self-control while formal treatment progresses.

Develop Positive Rituals

Ritual is a way to provide predictability and routine as well as an opportunity to work through conflicts and losses.

Previously, we have spoken of ritual in connection with compulsive behaviors. For example, someone with anorexia nervosa may cut up her food into a precise number of pieces each time she has a meal and arrange them in a neat geometric pattern on the plate. Such ritual has a magical quality and is designed to ward off misfortune.

Ritual can also be constructive and help guide us through our daily lives. Many rituals are automatic and are performed without conscious attention. In a classic *All in the Family* episode, Archie and Meathead argue over the virtues of putting on "a sock and a sock, and a shoe and a shoe" versus "a sock and a shoe, and a sock and a shoe." Each believes deeply that his way is the only right way.

With ritual, there are at least some things we can always depend on to be the same. In religious services, we hear the same hymns over and over, week after week, and year after year, so they acquire a comforting familiarity that reaches deeply inside. The music may connect us with our own childhood, with others around us, and with timeless traditions. For some people, unfortunately, the religion of their youths is not so comforting. Rather, it represents the pretense and hypocrisy of abusive adults.

Ritual provides a sense of continuity over time in a world that often feels chaotic and disconnected. It provides a connectedness with other people and a sense of belonging. Whether it is our deepest personal beliefs or how we put on our shoes and socks, ritual builds a foundation for personal identity.

Twelve-step support groups provide a ritualized approach to recovery, while offering kinship with thousands of others who have walked the same path.

Ritual also helps guide us through the losses and changes that are inevitable in life. Grief over the death of a loved one is a long process that unfolds over years. Ritual brings us together with other mourners at the funeral and permits a final good-bye. Ritual may later mark the anniversaries of the death and keep us aware of the emotional significance of the day. Without these conscious reminders, we might be at the mercy of powerful feelings without understanding their origin.

Talk to Your Therapist

It is important for your therapist to know to what extent you are in control of your impulses. If you are in danger and need help in keeping safe, you should be direct about your needs and willing to consider whatever interventions or safeguards are offered. You and your therapist will work toward understanding the origins of your impulses so that you may better control them.

Talk to Yourself

When you are in crisis, your thoughts may become fragmented. You may be unable to recall strategies you have learned during times of clearer thinking. Recorded messages to yourself can help you to refocus at such times. These messages could be as simple as a few key words carried in a well-marked envelope in your purse. A red envelope for emergencies would be particularly suitable and would remind you it is there.

Audiotaped or videotaped messages can be a powerful tool for recalling ideas. Such messages in your own voice can reconnect you with moments of clarity and insight. Your own healthy side is, after all, your most credible source of information about you and your best counselor.

If you follow these basic strategies, your life will begin to develop consistency from day to day. You will no longer react helter-skelter to randomly changing surroundings. Your mood will no longer be ruled by physical stress or unsatisfied needs for food, sleep, companionship, or drugs. Your life will no longer be lived in scattered fragments, but will acquire at last a sense of enduring wholeness.

*S*ara had been out of touch with Mark for several years. When they had last made contact, he was living in New York, unemployed and still drinking heavily. He had already been married and divorced twice and had one son from his first marriage. After leaving his parents' home, Mark had no stomach for conflict. Whenever the fighting began in his marriages, which it inevitably did because of his drinking, Mark simply left. He had left his son behind with some regret, but in his sober moments, he deeply believed that he would only have brought him pain.

Unbeknownst to Sara, Mark was also now well into recovery. Living in a suburb of Boston, he had stopped drinking for more than two years and was still attending AA meetings regularly. He was working days as a salesman in a downtown Boston department store and taking courses at Boston University at night. He hoped to eventually become an addictions counselor.

As chaotic as his life had been before, Mark now attended scrupulously to a healthy lifestyle. Not only had he stopped drinking, but he had also stopped smoking. He had become a vegetarian and was running on a daily basis. He was training to run in the Boston Marathon the following spring. Sleep was the one area of his life he still neglected. Fortunately, he required very little.

What brought Mark the most satisfaction, though, was the renewal of his relationship with his son, Joshua, who was now ten. After passing the first anniversary of his recovery, he had decided that he no longer posed a threat to Joshua's security and celebrated by contacting him. His ex-wife acknowledged the changes that he had undertaken and was happy for him, cooperating fully with his efforts to see his son. He now had regular visitation, including a full month during summer vacation. After an initial period of awkwardness, during which Mark explained as best he could the reason for his prolonged absence, they became fast friends.

During his recovery, Mark thought often of Sara. She had been the angrier of the two when they had last parted. Since making amends with those whom he had hurt was one of the steps in his recovery program, Mark wanted very much to contact her. But each time he would pick up the telephone, he recalled the venom in her voice at their last meeting and put the handset back in its cradle. Once he wrote her a long letter, but it ended up sitting on his dresser for months until he finally threw it away.

Now Sara also thought about contacting Mark, but she had no idea where to find him. She contacted his second wife, who had also lost touch. Sara had long ago lost touch with Mark's first wife and with her nephew. She believed that Mark was the missing link in her recovery and became obsessed with finding him. Through her relationship with Tom, she understood that Mark's animosity toward their father was more than just adolescent rebellion. She suspected that he, too, had been a victim of their father's drinking.

Then one night Sara called me at three in the morning. She spoke with a mixture of excitement and distress. She had struggled all evening with urges to cut herself, she told me, and managed to resist them. There followed another flashback of particular intensity.

"This one was different," she explained. "I have to see you right away."

17

When You Are Angry

When angry, count ten before you speak;
if very angry, an hundred.
THOMAS JEFFERSON

When angry, count four; when very angry, swear.
MARK TWAIN

Anger is the forbidden emotion. An infant imag-
ines that his angry feelings will destroy his caretakers.
The toddler's rage is met with the disapproval of impa-
tient adults. As children, we are chastised to control
our angry feelings, often by adults who are themselves
responding angrily.

Anger and rage are feelings charged with energy.
The combination of emotion and energy is a potentially destructive force. The bursts of energy that fuel
anger, however, can also be used constructively, just
as the destructive force of lightning can be harnessed
to run an engine. Anger can be the force behind solving problems, creating works of art, or bringing about
social change.

Anger is connected strongly with powerlessness.
We feel angry when we are hurt or frustrated and are

unable to do anything about it. If someone is responsible for our pain or deprivation, they become the object of our anger. If we are responsible, anger may be turned to guilt. If nobody is responsible and we cannot find anyone to blame, we may become angry at God or at the world at large.

Anger may arise simply from current pain. But if we have been hurt badly enough in the past, the pain may linger to resurface again and again together with renewed anger. If you are borderline, you are likely to have suffered unbearable pain and helplessness as a child, and the intensity of your rage can be fraught with danger. It can result in self-injury or suicide, aggression toward others, or emotional disintegration. When rage is turned toward family and friends, relationships are at risk. When feelings become too intense, dissociation or "numbing out" may occur so that no feelings are accessible.

Controlling the destructive force of anger is not the same as stuffing it inside. We can approach an immediate emotional crisis first by separating the energy from the feeling and discharging it. We can then take steps to understand and express the underlying emotion constructively.

Energy may be discharged by diverting it to vigorous exercise, competitive sports, or physical labor. Not only can exercising to exhaustion defuse rage, it can also have a mood-elevating effect of its own, particularly when done with regularity. Activities that permit controlled aggression, such as hitting a punching bag or martial arts training, may be particularly helpful in channeling anger. The latter also provides exposure to positive ritual and discipline and development of self-confidence, self-esteem, and security.

Reclaiming power is the key to taming anger. This begins with clarifying the root of our powerlessness. What form of pain or loss threatens us? How do we feel helpless? Who is in a position to restore us with power?

One type of threat to security is an imbalance between power and responsibility. If we feel responsible for the outcome of a situation, but lack the power to bring it about, guilt or anger may result. Clarifying appropriate limits of responsibility may resolve the dilemma. An extreme example of this is the inappropriate feeling of responsibility that children often feel for their own victimization.

Once the sources of anger have been identified, assertive expression of feelings or wishes may help to restore control. This may simply mean expressing a feeling about the specific actions of another person together with a request for corrective action. While others will not always respond by meeting your needs, expressing them can itself be empowering.

When the object of your anger is unavailable, assertive expression can still be achieved by journaling, writing letters, role play, or other forms of creative expression. If you are so inclined, this may also take the form of art, music, or poetry. Dragons may be slain in our hearts with abandon and without risk.

Power is meaningful when it serves to ensure our own security and well-being. Revenge is an illusion of power that often robs us of real control. When we seek revenge, we no longer have our own best interests at heart.

Imagine that you are in an ice cream parlor and have to choose between two flavors: your favorite and one you despise. Imagine further that your feelings are linked by ESP to your worst enemy's and that whatever you experience, he will, too. How would you choose? If you decide to punish your enemy, you will punish yourself as well. You will give up the freedom to choose what is best for you.

When you let others "push your buttons," you also give away power. You give them the power to trigger powerful emotions at will. Once you are aware of your own reactions, you can disconnect the buttons so they no longer work. When buttons don't work, people eventually stop pushing them. When that happens, you have claimed meaningful power.

Anger is often a trigger for drinking or drug use. This is

another way to numb feelings. Unfortunately, alcohol and drugs first anesthetize the parts of the brain that control judgment and self-restraint. Intoxication is another way to give your power away.

You may find that no matter what you do, you cannot let go of your anger. You may even discover that as you contemplate giving up anger, you feel anxious, even panicky. Your anger may have become the only enduring aspect of your shattered identity. To give up your victimhood would be like giving up a lifelong companion. Such losses must be grieved. And identity must then grow around a new, healthier core.

You may feel like Celia, who was repeatedly molested by an uncle as a small child. At forty-three, injured in an accident and wracked by chronic pain, Celia seethed inside with rage at her distant and aging uncle.

"I can never forget or forgive," Celia would say, "because if I do, he's won." Celia could not understand that by nurturing her ancient anger she continued to give her uncle power.

Celia's anger was also a potent force behind her chronic pain. Without current pain and misery, there would be little to justify her outrage. Pain had become another part of the fragile identity to which she clung.

If you were victimized, you have likely been robbed of the self-image you once possessed. This may have included innocence, security, the capacity to trust others, the capacity to trust yourself, and dignity. In place of these feelings came shame, guilt, and anger.

Healing is not something that occurs between you and your abuser. It is a process that occurs within you when you part with shame, guilt, and anger and reclaim what you once lost. Only then can you become free to develop healthy relationships with the people presently around you.

I arranged to meet Sara in my office first thing in the morning before my usual office schedule began. She was waiting for me at the door. She looked troubled and fatigued. Neither of us had been back to sleep.

"I had a new flashback," Sara began as soon as she sat down. "I feel so confused and guilty, I don't know how I'm ever going to live with myself again."

One night shortly after her sixth birthday, Sara heard her daddy coming up the stairs. She began trembling with fear, but he never came to get her. This time he went to her four-year-old brother's room. She listened to him clatter down the stairs and heard the same familiar scene unfold.

From then on, her daddy would sometimes come for her and sometimes for Mark. She would lay very still and pray each time that it would be Mark's turn. When she heard the door to her brother's room, she felt the same momentary surge of relief that she had felt whenever the gun fell away, followed by waves of nausea as the distant scene played out.

Once, the gun went off and Sara imagined Mark lying bleeding and motionless on the floor. But her father had shot at the furniture to show her mother he meant business. Sara had been frantic. When she heard Mark come back up the stairs to go back to bed, she burst into tears of relief. But she was so ashamed of her own cowardice that she could not let him see her that night. Sara and Mark never discussed these episodes, perhaps because talking about them would make them more real or perhaps because of the guilt each suffered the times that they were spared.

"How could I have wished such a thing on him?" Sara lamented. "He was so little and helpless."

"You were little and helpless, too." I replied.

"But I was his big sister. Wasn't I supposed to protect him?"

"How?"

"I don't know," Sara answered, shaking her head sadly. "I really have no idea at all."

Sara's guilt was similar to that of a concentration camp survivor who has watched others perish. Worse than the guilt, though, was the shame she experienced for having wished the horror upon him. To Sara at age six, simply wishing it made her responsible for it happening. She could not understand then that they were both equally helpless victims, neither having the power to influence their father's senseless acts or random choices. Neither could she understand that wishing for her own survival was not the same as wishing for Mark to be punished.

Now Sara understood why Mark had so hated her daddy and she could at last forgive him for it. She also understood for the first time that their estrangement had begun long before they were teenagers. It started with the silence they shared as children about the atrocities they had suffered.

Sara's guilt had served to maintain the fiction that somehow she had the power to alter events and escape the pain. It protected her from having to acknowledge her total helplessness. As Sara began to let go of the shame and guilt that she had carried all those years, she felt overwhelmed by the enormity of that helplessness and her rage at her father was redoubled. Not only had he terrorized them all, but he had divided them with guilt, shame, and anger so that they were each left to suffer alone.

Sara was now left to deal with her terrible rage. As she sat in my office, she recalled for the first time her trips to the cemetery. The first had followed Jonathan's story of the little boy who had been shot and had occurred prior to any conscious recollection of her own betrayal. The story had triggered the deeply buried terror that had accompanied the sound of her father's gun. She was drawn then to her father's grave by a force that she had no way of understanding. By the second visit, she had become aware of the betrayal, but not of its depth.

Now I suggested that Sara plan another visit, this time not in mindless flight but with a purpose. First she was to write a letter to her father, which she would read at the graveside. She might choose to go alone or perhaps with Jonathan if she felt willing to let him this far into her life. This would be an opportunity not only to heal old wounds, but perhaps also to begin repairing the damage she had done to her present-day relationships. Sara brought the letter to her next session.

18

Intimacy
Managing Emotional Distance

We should be careful to get out of an experience only the wisdom that is in it—and stop there; lest we be like the cat that sits down on a hot stove lid. She will never sit down on a hot stove lid again—and that is well; but also she will never sit down on a cold one any more.

MARK TWAIN

Imagine looking in a mirror. As you peer closer and closer, the details of the image in the mirror become clearer. Now imagine your nose touching the surface of the mirror and merging with the nose on the other side until the image in the mirror reaches out and yanks you all the way inside.

If you are borderline, relationships may feel a lot like this renegade mirror. The other person provides a screen on which you reflect features of your own image as you struggle to define who you are. As you move closer in the relationship the image sharpens, but when you move too close, the image begins to blur and finally engulfs you. When relationships are distant or nonexistent, it is like looking in the mirror and seeing only emptiness.

If you are borderline, your relationships may be

short-lived and passionate. You are either "in love" or "in hate." Your involvement with the other person is sustained by the passion of either feeling. Once the passion subsides, at the point in a relationship when true intimacy usually begins to form, you become bored and move on to a new object of passion.

As your relationships persist, instead of deepening concern and communication, there ensues a struggle for control. The arena of this often violent struggle may include time, money, sex, fidelity, spiritual beliefs, children, or physical and emotional distance. The centerpiece of the struggle is the threat of abandonment.

During the struggle, you may be physically or sexually abused. In your attempts to regain power, you may resort to emotional blackmail, with threats ranging from sexual distance to self-injury or suicide. Such blackmail may bring you considerable momentary power, but at the expense of your becoming the object of intense resentment or rage. Your victims are likely to feel like hostages and eventually strike back or flee.

Despite the pain you experience in relationships, you continue to search for the one that will be different. And each new love will shine for a time. The passion of your encounters with others serves as a momentary distraction from the profound feelings of loneliness that constantly haunt you. You need to be loved because you have not yet learned how to feel comfortable and secure in your own company. You seek someone who will fill the emptiness inside you rather than an equal partner with whom to share life's experiences and responsibilities. Once you think you have found such a person, you struggle to avoid rejection.

Despite this intense need to be loved, formidable barriers keep you from allowing anyone too near. You may have been hurt in the past by others you have trusted. Your inability to trust would be particularly strong if betrayals began with your earliest childhood experiences. The prospect of love and an awareness of danger would then go hand in hand.

Deepening of love requires that love be returned. If you feel empty inside, you are likely to feel that you have little to give or that any effort to give will leave you completely drained.

Emotional closeness intensifies the possibility of being discovered unworthy and being rejected. Feelings of unworthiness may be connected with shameful secrets that you bear or with a deeper sense of incompleteness. Most of all, you may fear boring others, which is a counterpoint to your own struggle to avoid the vacuum of boredom that allows despair to infiltrate. Closeness raises the emotional stakes if you are eventually rejected.

Finally, intimacy threatens the delicate balance of your identity. As with the image in the mirror, you develop a fleeting sense of self within a relationship, borrowing and trying on aspects of the other person. With intimacy, however, comes the threat of being engulfed completely and losing any sense of separate identity.

There is no simple way to avoid the chaos that relationships hold for you. With heightened awareness, however, you may be able to control some of the damage that your impulsive reactions can wreak. Identifying the feelings behind the behavior and connecting feelings with the degree of closeness you feel in key relationships can help restore your power to choose what you do. Here are some suggestions for controlling your impulsive reactions.

Monitor Emotional Distance

Draw a five-inch line across a sheet of paper. Think about your most important current relationship: Consider the extreme left as feeling totally alone and the extreme right as feeling thoroughly smothered. Make a mark representing how you feel in the relationship today. Mark the limits of your comfort zone. Draw a new line each day and mark it the same way. This will provide a running graph of how you perceive the rhythm of the relationship.

You can monitor more than one relationship at a time and more than one kind of relationship. You might even try using a graph of this type to track your relationship with your therapist.

Think Before You Act

Keep track of your most destructive behaviors. When the impulse first arises, try to identify how you feel. Then examine how the feeling is related to the emotional distance you feel in important relationships. For example, you may feel sad or angry when you believe someone important to you is about to abandon you.

Next, consider the most likely outcome of the behavior. Is it likely to increase the distance in your relationship or to bring you closer? How does this compare with your perceived need for distance at the time? How does the probable long-term outcome compare with the anticipated short-term outcome?

Yvonne was a twenty-five-year-old model in an eight-month-long relationship with her boyfriend, Damon. Over several weeks, Damon began showing increasing interest in a twenty-year-old colleague of Yvonne's. Increasingly fearful that he would leave her, Yvonne took an overdose of drugs within an hour of Damon's expected arrival from work.

Horrified and feeling responsible for this close call, Damon appeared at her bedside in the hospital and pledged his eternal devotion. Once the initial shock wore off, however, he became more horrified at the prospect of repeating this scene over and over and took the opportunity of her admission to a psychiatric hospital to leave her.

Identify Feelings

Behind drastic actions lie desperate feelings. When you hold back action, you will inevitably experience intense negative feelings. At first, you will be aware only of feeling awful. When you look more closely, however, you may be able to distinguish sadness, terror, rage, guilt, envy, or humiliation. These emotions may provide additional clues to the danger that the action was intended to protect against. Although sadness, for example, may go along with feeling abandoned, guilt is more likely to indicate excessive closeness, a relationship that is treading on forbidden ground.

By getting feelings into the open, you can test their validity. Sometimes a trivial event can trigger a chain of fantasy, with a conclusion that has a life of its own. Once the assumptions behind emotions are clarified, the evidence that supports them can be weighed fairly.

Talk Effectively

Communication is the cornerstone of a sound relationship. When you communicate only through action, the messages can become severely distorted. Action tends to provoke action, equally garbling the incoming message. Words are essential to accurate communication.

Even words must be chosen carefully if the picture that forms in your partner's mind is to match your own idea. You may suggest, for example, going out to dinner and your partner enthusiastically agrees. You were thinking of a candlelight dinner in a cozy restaurant, but he is already on the telephone while you are dressing, calling two other couples to meet you at the sports bar down the street. The evening is destroyed with a fight before it ever begins.

When you talk and listen, you have the best chance to correct misperceptions about the other person or his intentions. When your language includes feeling-words, you communicate most completely about yourself. This gives your partner the best possible opportunity to meet your needs.

Make Contracts

Contracts are the ultimate means to clarify expectations. Most businesses would not think of dealing with other businesses without having agreements in writing. And yet the most important transactions of our lives are bound with the flimsiest communications.

Contracts can provide predictability and structure where only chaos once reigned. You may include in your contracts provisions about time, money, sex, or any area in which conflict might arise. You may provide for how, together, you will handle lapses in self-control on either partner's part. You may provide for daily times to talk, specific times to play together, and scheduled time apart. You may provide for times to revise and renew your contracts. You may even delineate how to dissolve the relationship if either partner should choose to do so and on what grounds this might occur.

With honest contracting, opportunities for emotional blackmail can be minimized, weakening the forces that drive your most destructive behaviors.

Diversify Your Relationships

Lovers provide only one kind of relationship that contributes to self-fulfillment. Relationships with family members, enduring friendships, and close working relationships all are part of a well-balanced life. The more meaningful relationships you enjoy, the less power any single relationship has to destroy your world. The richness of your relationships also enhances what you bring to each of them.

To consider identity without a framework of relationships would be like examining an elegant artifact without knowing anything about the culture within which it was created. While such an object may have aesthetic appeal, it would have limited meaning. Continuity of identity means not only consistency of values, attitudes, and feelings over time, but the interweaving of your life in a stable way within a tapestry of relationships and culture.

When Sara visited her father's grave, Jonathan was by her side holding her hand. Here is what she read:

Dear Daddy,

Why did you die before I had a chance to tell you all that is in my heart? You can never know the intensity of the pain you caused me then and for the rest of my life. Now I am ready to let go of my pain and begin to live.

I always thought you loved me. I find it unbearable to know that even for a moment you could use me and endanger me and frighten me the way you did. If you truly loved me, I imagine that you suffered terrible guilt and shame over the years before you died. I wonder if you remembered even a fraction of what you did to all of us? I wonder if you had any more idea than I why Mark was so embittered toward you?

What has been hardest for me was that for so many years I adored you. You really were such a good daddy for all the years I could remember before the shadows of those dark, dark early years intruded into my life.

When I discovered what you had done to me, to all of us, I was robbed even of my happier memories of you. Now I hope to reclaim those memories, which have been stolen from me twice.

Daddy, there is something important that I have never told you. Do you remember when I was a sophomore in college how things between us suddenly changed? I was too ashamed to face you because I had had an abortion and I was afraid you'd be able to tell and be terribly disillusioned. Well, I guess disillusionment goes with the territory when you really love someone. You accept them as they are, flaws and all.

I know that you were an alcoholic and that the liquor poisoned your brain. It made you think horrible thoughts and it *made you do horrible things. I understand the hold it had on you because I am an alcoholic, too.*

Still, I hate that you let it go on so long without getting help and that you allowed it to hurt us so badly. You were as much a victim as we were.

Well, I am ready to stop being a victim, and I am ready for my family to stop being victimized by my behavior. I am worthwhile, and I deserve to be treated well by others and most of all, by myself. With this letter, I am finally burying the pain with you.

When you died I turned my back and couldn't say good-bye. Now at last I can. Daddy, I love you very much, and I'll miss you. Goodbye.

                    Your daughter,
                    Sara

When Sara finished reading the letter, she turned to Jonathan and saw tears that matched her own quietly streaming down his cheeks. Then Jonathan picked up the shovel they had brought and began to dig a small hole next to the headstone while Sara carried over the crape myrtle they brought to plant there. When the hole was dug, she placed the letter in it before planting the tree. They took turns shoveling in the soil until the hole was filled.

The plant had been Jonathan's idea. It was fitting that something beautiful should grow from this soil. They would return year after year to watch it grow and flower. Sara never felt closer to Jonathan or more loving. She felt wedded to him for the first time in their marriage. They gently patted down the freshly turned soil. Then together they went home.

19

Bewitched, Bothered, and Bewildered

Living with a Borderline Person

My dear, I don't give a damn.
RHETT BUTLER
Gone with the Wind
MARGARET MITCHELL

If you are in a relationship with someone with BPD, you are likely to feel bewildered, frustrated, angry, frightened, bewitched, and helpless. You may sometimes wish to flee, but can't, perhaps because of the wonderful magnetism that draws you to her, or perhaps because you feel her fragility and fear that she would not survive your loss.

You were attracted to her, not because of who she was, but because of her uncanny ability to be whomever you needed her to be. Without a clear identity of her own, she locked in her radar on yours, and she became a mirror for those qualities you yearned for in yourself.

You fell in love with the person you were when you were with her. In the beginning, you most likely felt admired, adored, and deeply needed. With her black-

and-white view of the world, she cast special qualities upon you and basked in their light, bewitching you both.

Now you find the mirror reflecting the darker side of yourself. She is director of the piece. When she casts you as a villain, you may feel and even act villainous. At worst, you may participate in recreating her victimization by becoming physically, sexually, or emotionally abusive. At best you may feel yourself a victim, an object of rage held hostage by self-destructive acts for which she holds you to blame.

You have also become aware of the terror of intimacy that may have lain behind a facade of seductive sensuality. As you have become more involved with each other, sex likely has become more difficult or nonexistent. It may be particularly drenched in conflict if she has been sexually abused.

If you are reading this chapter, you have probably already decided to hang on for the rest of the ride. You can expect it to be bumpy and unpredictable. What follows are some basic principles for survival.

Maintain Boundaries

You are responsible for your own actions. You are not responsible for hers. While you cannot always deflect the rage that is directed at you, you can avoid retaliation. If you struggle with impulses to strike back, the chapters on controlling impulses and anger may help you learn how to contain them. Remember who owns the rage. Remember, too, that its origins long predate your arrival on the scene.

Communicate Feelings

Trouble occurs when painful feelings are acted out. Tell her how you feel and identify which of her actions led to the feeling. Focus on your own emotional response rather than passing judgment on her behavior. Not only will this help you respond more rationally, but it will provide her an opportunity to talk about her own feelings rather than to act upon them.

Make Contracts

As you gain experience with the kinds of conflicts that arise between you, you may be able to anticipate the most likely problems that lie ahead. Together, develop a plan for addressing them. It would be particularly helpful to define clearly what your role will be if she threatens suicide or self-injury. This will help prevent you from rewarding such behavior with special attention.

Maintain Respect for One Another

Appreciate the human struggle behind the behaviors that so enrage you at times. Learn what you can about the history of her struggle, and share what you can about yours. Developing an interest in each other's backgrounds can help you both develop a clearer sense of your individual identities and create appropriate boundaries in your relationship.

Be a Partner in Therapy

Couples therapy is an important component of treatment. It presents an opportunity to examine your interactions with each other and to discuss your own reactions. It also offers a chance to discuss any acting out that has occurred and to develop strategies for preventing it in the future. The therapist's role in addressing self-destructive behaviors should be clearly defined.

If you have just picked up this book and turned directly to this chapter, going back and reading the book from the beginning will give you a headstart in understanding her turmoil. Reading each chapter together and discussing it as you go along can open up your dialogue with each other.

Remember Who the Therapist Is

Your role in this relationship is as partner, companion, and friend. You are not responsible for providing a cure. Your role is limited to providing a respectful and hopefully loving atmosphere in which emotional growth can flourish.

Develop Your Own Support System

Having others with whom you can discuss your feelings and reactions may help keep you grounded in reality and enable you to maintain control. Therapy is one possible source of support. Support groups may be particularly helpful. Codependency groups address many of the problems you face in relating to someone who is out of control. There also may be specific groups in your community for people in relationships like yours.

If you are patient, you may take part in an exciting process of discovery as the pieces of a beautiful creation are fitted together one by one, and it takes shape before your eyes. Your relationship may then become a featured room in an elaborate museum within which her growing identity can flourish.

*J*onathan was no stranger to chaos. He was the oldest of four children, with three younger sisters. His father was a long-distance truck driver who was sometimes away for weeks at a time. His mother had been a waitress who continued to work until she was seven months into her second pregnancy. When she had to take time off because of problems with her blood pressure, she never went back. A child of an alcoholic father, she was herself addicted to tranquilizers and pain pills. Many times Jonathan had to feed and look after his younger siblings while she was passed out on the couch.

Once when he was eight, he came home from school and she appeared more still than usual. In place of the usual heavy breathing of her drugged sleeps, her breathing was shallow. He could not arouse her and called the rescue squad, which brought her to the hospital where her stomach was pumped. Jonathan never knew for sure whether the overdose was accidental or she had tried to kill herself. From then on he became her guardian, sometimes hiding the pills when he thought she'd had too many and always watching her closely when he was home. He always feared that one day he would come home from school and find her dead.

When Jonathan was fourteen, his mother developed breast cancer. When the lump was first found, she stuck her head in the sand and took more pills. By the time she had the biopsy, it was the size of a golf ball. Within a year she was dead. While she was dying, his father gave up trucking and took a job in a factory so that he could be with his family. By this time, however, he was already tired and defeated from years of struggling to support his family and putting up with his wife's addictions.

Jonathan left home at sixteen and went to work as a hospital orderly while finishing high school at night. He enjoyed the medical setting, believing that here, at least, people got well and things weren't so hopeless. When he finished high school, he went on to train as an emergency medical technician. This held special appeal because the excitement of the rescues stood in contrast to the moribund atmosphere in which he grew up. But try as he might, Jonathan was not an adventurer. At his core, he was responsible, conservative, and practical.

It was color and vibrance that had attracted him to both his wives. His first wife turned out to be self-indulgent and reckless. Still, Jonathan had remained hopeful about their marriage until its demise was undeniable. With Sara there seemed to be more substance. For all her acting out, Jonathan always believed in her basic goodness and that she cared for him and their children.

As tolerant as Jonathan was, though, he stayed on guard against another betrayal. He would not stand for another. abandonment. So he had a great deal of trouble understanding Sara's episodes of lost time and her late nights. When she had returned from the second trip to the cemetery roughed up and grass stained, all he could think of was that she had had a sexual tryst. He never considered other alternatives, even the possibility that she might have been raped.

This was Jonathan's most significant weakness, one that almost led him to leave her early in treatment. But he never voiced his suspicions. After the beating, Sara came clean about the flirtations and teasing that had led up to it. This, Jonathan took well, and he was able to be supportive when she most needed him. He sensed the rage behind this behavior and somehow understood that it had nothing to do with faithlessness and did not threaten their relationship.

The most frightening event for Jonathan in the course of Sara's treatment was her fast. Since it came on the heels of a tirade that seemed to be directed at him, he was personally hurt by it and somehow felt responsible for it. As she became more and more emaciated, resembling his mother during her terminal illness, he became terrified of losing her this way. One way or another, the women in his life always abandoned him.

Jonathan particularly shined as a father. During all the times Sara was hospitalized or otherwise absent, Jonathan had kept the children's lives as normal as possible. He gave them plenty of opportunities to talk about their feelings when Sara was in crisis and to ask questions. Unfortunately, he had very few answers for them.

When they visited the cemetery together, Jonathan at last felt a part of Sara's life. For the first time since he had known her, she let him share in the fullness of her feelings. Only now did he realize that she never had before. And for the first time in several years, he was not afraid of losing her. For him, too, this was their wedding day.

20

Beyond Survival

Is There A Cure?

*"Real isn't how you are made," said the Skin Horse.
"It's a thing that happens to you. When a child loves
you for a long, long time, not just to play with,
REALLY loves you, then you become Real. It doesn't
happen all at once. You become. It takes a long time.
Generally, by the time you are Real, most of your hair
has been loved off, and your eyes drop out and you get
loose in the joints and very shabby. But these things
don't matter at all, because once you are Real you can't
be ugly, except to people who don't understand."*

The Velveteen Rabbit
MARGERY WILLIAMS

T reatment can be stormy. During long-term treatment, many crises can occur, some life threatening. Hospitalization may be needed to cope with moments of despair. It is worth it? Does treatment bring change? What can you expect at the end of the journey through the inner workings of your emotional life? Can you acquire the lasting belief in yourself that is part of being "Real"?

Wounds heal in several stages. First, the wound is open, vulnerable to infection or reinjury. Later, a scab forms. If the scab is disturbed, bleeding may recur and

159

part of the healing process starts over. When healing is complete, the site of the wound is still visible for a time. Later, there is a scar, which may be faint or prominent. It may itch sometimes and remind you it is there, but it no longer commands your attention. Some scars are thin and vulnerable to new injury. Others are thick and tougher than the surrounding tissues.

Emotional healing is similar. Wounds can heal, but they usually remind you where they have been. You may remain vulnerable in some areas that have healed, while you develop unusual wisdom and strength in others. The very pattern of your scars will become part of your developing sense of a consistent self.

Early in the journey, you will wish to erase the past as if the painful, shameful experiences never happened. As you discover that this is impossible, you will learn instead to make peace with it, so that the past may fade into the background and no longer dominate your experience.

At the end of the journey is trust and forgiveness. If you are treated by a therapist who values you even through times of conflict and disappointment, who values your safety and well-being, and who helps you to grow in self-confidence, responsibility, and self-respect, then trust will follow. Establishing a sustained, trusting relationship that is tolerant of transgressions, but is never exploited or betrayed, will enable you to trust others and yourself.

Trust and forgiveness are inseparable. At the heart of trust is an enduring faith in the goodness of another person even when he disappoints you. At the heart of self-respect is an enduring faith in your own goodness even when you disappoint yourself. When such faith is established, there comes a reassuring sense of soundness in yourself and the world. This is the basis of a stable, multidimensional identity.

With trust and forgiveness come the capacity to be alone peacefully and to be with others. Emotional intimacy is built on mutual trust, respect, and investment in mutual growth. With intimacy comes the opportunity to reclaim your sexuality.

As you leave your black-and-white existence and learn to appreciate the many-faceted qualities of others, your early impressions will grow more accurate and you will place your trust more wisely. As your boundaries become more clearly defined, you will detect more quickly when others violate them. When the wounds are healed, the sharks will no longer circle.

W hen Sara came to her next session, she reported a dream. In the dream she is riding on a motorcycle, her hair streaming freely in the wind. She is heading home via a new route. She approaches a building, a skyscraper. From a distance, it looks dismal, plain, and granite. As she nears it, however, she is suddenly struck by its beauty. Hues of azure streak through the marbled stone. Glistening crystal protrudes in an irregular outline along the sides.

She is not in a hurry and stops to look closer. She goes to park the motorcycle. She finds all the parking spaces filled with presents people have left there while they shop. When she is closer to the building, she notices that it stands in the middle of an unfinished square of plain cement and asphalt. There are a few potholes. It needs to be landscaped.

By now Sara was a seasoned interpreter of her own dreams and proceeded to teach me what this one meant.

"I think," she began, "that the building is me . . . my life. The distant view is how I used to look at my life. The closer view represents the richness and beauty I have discovered within me during treatment. It is the present. The presents in the street tell me that the present now holds good things for me. And the square around the building reminds me that the work is not over. There is always more growing to do. The building's pretty solid," Sara laughed, "now I guess it's time to tend to the landscaping."

It is so often hard to tell when the work of therapy is done. It does not end merely with the unearthing of deeply buried secrets. For as we have seen, it is hard to know just when all the crucial secrets have been discovered. The memories must also be understood in new ways so that painful feelings can be put to rest. Even then the treatment is not done. There must also be a decision to use this newfound understanding in order to live differently.

As a therapist, I look for signs that tell me real change has occurred. The abandonment of symptoms is one such sign. For

Sara, this meant staying sober, no longer hurting or starving herself, and being freed from the horror of flashbacks to a time long gone. The capacity to enjoy richly intimate relationships is another sign. Sara and Jonathan had certainly come a long way in finding love. Sara did locate Mark, and they also began to enjoy a loving relationship with each other.

Sometimes we are graced with a sign that uniquely confirms that the end of treatment is at hand. Such was Sara's last dream and her interpretation of it. It told me that she had learned enough about self-exploration that she was ready to continue this lifelong quest on her own. It told me, too, that she had realistic expectations about what was yet to come, that she was prepared to accept the imperfections in herself and the ones she loved. This was her parting gift to me.

21

Am I My Patient's Keeper?

The Dilemma of Treating People with Borderline Personality Disorder

Life is short, and the Art long; the occasion fleeting; experience fallacious, and judgment difficult. The physician must not only be prepared to do what is right himself, but also to make the patient, the attendants, and externals cooperate.

Aphorisms
HIPPOCRATES

This chapter is addressed to therapists. It is intended not as a manual for treating patients with BPD, but to highlight the emotional struggles facing anyone who undertakes the task. It is like an archaeologist's guide, not to the work of unearthing treasures, but to the terrain that must be traveled in the process.

The most challenging task of treating patients with BPD is defining and maintaining clear boundaries between you and your patient. This makes sense, given the developmental task of separation and individuation with which patients are struggling. Boundary definition begins at the beginning of treatment.

The boundary of responsibility for your patient's

behavior is perhaps the most difficult to establish and defend. You may spend one hour a week with your patient, yet assume responsibility for behavior that occurs during the remaining 167 hours. This behavior may include suicidal acts, self-mutilation, self-starvation, drug or alcohol abuse and its consequences, acts of aggression, and illegal activities. Your patient may even become responsible for the serious injury or death of others.

The potential for such disasters can result in many sleepless nights for therapists. Many forces can create a powerful impression that you can and should control your patient's behavior. Your patient may herself view you as an omnipotent protector, much as toddlers expect protection as they explore their world helter-skelter. This may play into your rescue fantasies as you willingly take on this treacherous role.

The legal system tends to hold treating professionals responsible for outcomes. An assumption of the legal system is that bad outcomes, particularly if unexpected, mean bad treatment. Clearly adverse outcomes such as suicide or serious self-injury leave you vulnerable to litigation, which can be devastating to your life and career. Whether or not litigation occurs, most therapists suffer emotionally in the wake of such events as they second-guess their own decisions and actions.

Therapy, therefore, takes place in an environment that tugs at any tendency you may have to become codependent. This can turn you into an enabler of your patient's most dreaded acts as you take on responsibility for preventing them. You then, in effect, become a hostage to the treatment process. Such a serious misalliance undermines your capacity to be therapeutic and contradicts the treatment goal of helping your patient assume control of her destiny.

Treatment is a long-term commitment that, in order to work, requires both partners to be reasonably comfortable. The length of a thorough course of treatment may be comparable to the length of captivity of the longest-held hostages in Lebanon. If you too become a hostage, the ordeal can be very painful.

To make matters worse, family members desperate for rescue may have unrealistic expectations of your power and may become angry when they are disappointed. You may take the rap in a husband's eyes for his wife's erratic temperament. You may be blamed if the relationship becomes rocky or if she withdraws sexually in the midst of exploring earlier experiences with sexual abuse.

Your commitment to confidentiality adds fuel to the fire. Confidentiality is particularly crucial to treatment of patients with BPD, since trust is indispensable to their capacity to disclose and explore painful issues. It may prevent you from communicating directly with those who are closest to your patient. While your contract for treatment is with your patient, family members may assume a contract with themselves as well, particularly if they encouraged or initiated the treatment or if they pay for it.

Your patient may take advantage of confidentiality by blaming you for her acting out. Patients with BPD can be experts at pitting others against one another; they can place you in mortal combat with their families and lovers. This permits them to disavow their own angry feelings while they watch the conflict being played out before them.

As a therapist, therefore, you may become the object of blame and possible legal action from disgruntled family members and from disillusioned patients. Splitting predisposes borderline patients to sudden bursts of anger that may be accompanied by a wish for revenge. While these feelings are best verbalized in the course of treatment, they may instead be acted out or bring treatment to an abrupt halt.

Don't Become a Hostage

Your role is most stressful when there is an imbalance between power and responsibility. Stress can be reduced by defining clear limits of responsibility and tapping legitimate sources of power in the treatment relationship.

Defining realistic expectations is a critical early task of treatment. When patients have surgery, they receive detailed information about the risks of the procedure. Discussing the risks of psychotherapy would seem equally appropriate. A treatment contract is an excellent vehicle for disclosing risks and defining the limits of what you can control.

A dialogue with close family members early in treatment is also desirable. This can occur only with your patient's consent and participation in the discussion. It would include a similar disclosure of risk and an identification of the expected benefits of treatment. It would be an opportunity to predict some of the emotional reactions that family members experience when someone is in therapy. It would allow you to identify resources for emotional support and to provide references, such as *Lost in the Mirror*, for learning about what their loved one may be experiencing. It would be a time to negotiate the management of crises and to define how confidentiality will be handled.

Treatment Contracts

Contracts are an effective way to control the chaos that can occur in therapy and to preserve the alliance between you and your patient. A contract identifies the mutual goals of treatment and defines the responsibility of each participant in working toward those goals. Contracts emphasize that therapy is not something done to, but with, patients.

Contracts provide predictability for patients who have become accustomed to inconsistency in their relationships. They provide a reality base in a relationship prone to raging fantasy. They also provide for either party to be able to terminate the contract if the goals are not likely to be met. A typical treatment contract would include the following elements.

Statement of Goals

Both long-term and short-term goals should be identified. Long-term goals could be framed initially in terms of the criteria for BPD that each patient meets. For example, a contract for one patient might focus on control of self-destructive impulses; for another, on developing stable relationships; and for still another, on developing a stable pattern of identity. While more than one issue might be addressed, it is helpful to identify a problem that appears central to each patient's emotional pain.

Short-term goals would begin with changes that allow treatment to continue. Examples would include controlling suicidal impulses, developing a support system, and learning to manage time and money. It may be helpful in framing short-term goals to identify a target date for reaching each one.

Responsibility for Appointments
An appointment is actually a reservation for a chunk of your time. It should be understood that both of you will strive to be on time for the appointment. Your contract should spell out what will happen if either of you is late for an appointment or is unable to keep the appointment. It also should specify consequences for multiple missed appointments.

Responsibility for Payment
The cost of each session of specified length should be agreed upon in advance. The way in which payment is to be made and the timing of payments also should be specified. This would include responsibility for submitting insurance claims. If your bill is not paid at the time of your sessions, consequences should be defined for overdue payments.

This is of more than practical importance. Most of us assume that "you don't get something for nothing." This is a deeply held belief that governs our emotions and behavior. When we think we are getting away with something, our consciences often prevent us from getting anything good out of the situation.

As a resident, I tended, early in my training, to neglect the issue of payment. I deluded myself into thinking that the financial transaction was between the patient and the clinic and had nothing to do with me. This was partly related to my doubts that I had anything of value to offer my patients at that time. It also reflected my own fantasy that the help I offered was unselfishly given and in endless supply.

Annette had been in treatment for nearly a year. I had become frustrated and puzzled at her lack of progress. Each session was much like the one before, with little new material or any evidence of change. At the end of one session, she recalled a childhood memory in which she had taken one of her sister's dolls and had felt so guilty she could not enjoy playing with it.

When I heard the theme of getting away with a theft, I decided to check her account and discovered that she had never paid a penny toward her bill. I came to the next session armed with the bill and ready to confront her. She beat me to the punch by announcing at the start of the session that she had just paid her entire bill on the way in! This transaction provided a richness of associated experiences and fantasies that helped clarify her presenting problem. The remainder of her treatment unfolded over only eight more sessions to a successful conclusion.

The crucial influence of payment on the treatment experience is complicated today by the influence of third-party payments. In some cases, such as with Workers' Compensation, your patient may not be responsible for any part of the payment for her treatment. In other cases, her involvement may be minimal, and she may not be made financially responsible for missed sessions or other breaches of her contract. In these cases, it is particularly important for you and your patient to define alternative consequences for such breaches. Another risk of not paying for treatment is a subtle influence on motivation to conclude treatment. We tend to work a lot faster when the meter is ticking than when the ride is free.

Frequency of Sessions

The frequency of sessions, as well as any conditions for changing the frequency, should be decided early in treatment. This decision takes into account the severity of your patient's crisis and her risk of self-harm, whether or not she is taking medications that need monitoring, her time and financial constraints, and the goals of treatment. Frequent brief sessions might be appropriate at the height of a crisis, when risk is high, but she may not be ready to tolerate the emotional turmoil of exploring her past. Longer sessions might follow in which the goals of treatment would include learning about the origins of her feelings and behavior.

Once the frequency of sessions has been negotiated, it is vital for you to stay on schedule. It is particularly important to reevaluate your patient before represcribing medications, especially if suicide has been an issue.

Duration of Treatment
The length of treatment depends upon your goals. Crisis intervention might take just a few sessions. Resolving underlying emotional issues might take four or five years.

If you decide on limited, well-defined treatment goals, it is often useful to contract for an exact number of sessions. This helps keep the goal in sight and paces your work. In this case, you have agreed that, while there may be many problems, most will be left unsolved.

More commonly, treatment length is left open-ended without a clear-cut end point. In this case, it is helpful to contract for an initial term of treatment that is renewable like other contracts. This also provides an opportunity periodically to reevaluate goals.

Leaving treatment abruptly is one of the hazards of being borderline. Your patient will inevitably suffer disappointments in therapy. When she does not feel cared for in treatment, she is likely to walk away. Not only are most treatment impasses resolvable, they are usually opportunities for growth. The contract should specify that any decision to stop treatment would be discussed thoroughly before acting.

Emergencies

Emergencies are likely to be times of intense emotional pain in which your patient is at risk for behaving self-destructively. Your contract should describe how emergencies will be handled. If you are called, your interventions could include guidance in solving a problem, changes in medication, extra sessions, or hospitalization. Emergencies are exceptions to the usual course of treatment. If your patient "cries wolf" with frequent after-hours calls, your ability to help in a real emergency may be neutralized.

Provisions for hospitalization should be considered in advance. Hospitalization is usually reserved for emergencies such as risk of suicide. It might also be considered when signs of intense distress appear, such as frequent extra calls or shutting down communication. Other possible indicators for hospitalization include persistent depressed mood, feeling or acting out of control, and inability to maintain the treatment contract.

Often, mood and behavior changes leading to a crisis seriously disrupt routine, including the regular schedule for taking medications. This, in turn, leads to further deterioration of mood. Frequently missing medications, therefore, may be an indirect indicator of the need for hospitalization.

Suicide should be specifically addressed. Your patient should pledge in her contract to let you know promptly if she is considering suicide. It should be understood from the beginning that hospital admission will be mandatory if at any time during treatment she is unable to guarantee her safety at least until she is seen again.

Your contract may also contain special provisions to deal with risks accompanying each patient's particular symptoms and behavior. For example, if she has an eating disorder, hospitalization may be linked to a specified degree of weight loss or electrolyte imbalance.

Responsible Use of Medication

Most mood-altering medications can be risky if abused. Overdoses are common and too often fatal. Incomplete suicide attempts can result in permanent organ damage or brain damage. Some medications can be addictive when taken for more than a brief period of time. Some should not be combined with alcohol. Many can impair the ability to drive safely.

Many patients with BPD keep a "stash" of extra medications. This is a way of keeping open the option of suicide. It is a dangerous practice particularly for impulsive people. The stash may contain medications leftover from other doctors, medications prescribed by you that have been discontinued, and medications that have been accumulated from missed doses even when you have kept careful track of her needs. If a crisis involves angry feelings toward you, your patient may be particularly tempted out of vengeance to attempt suicide using the medications you prescribed.

It is a matter of life and death that your patient promises in her contract to use medications exactly as prescribed. The contract should require her to keep you accurately informed of all medications in her possession. If medications are no longer being used, she should destroy them or turn them in to you for disposal.

First of All, Do No Harm

If you are sincere in your efforts to help your patient and maintain her welfare as the focus of therapy, you are unlikely to cause her harm. If you exploit her in any way, however, you may retraumatize her and do irreparable harm. Respecting your patient's personal boundaries is crucial to the treatment process.

Sexual exploitation is certainly the most flagrant and damaging of the boundary violations a therapist can commit. More subtle seductive or manipulative behaviors can also be damaging. When a therapist seeks a patient's admiration in order to support his own self-esteem, the boundaries of therapy are violated. When a therapist imposes his own religious or political views on a patient, boundaries are violated.

Scrupulous honesty is the foundation on which good therapy is built. The requirement for honesty is mutual. Therapy reaches impasse whenever patients willfully withhold the truth. Therapy also flounders when therapists are deceitful or take unfair advantage of the power they have in the relationship.

During my training, I treated a young woman who was a talented poet. From time to time, she brought me packets of her work to read and eagerly awaited my reaction. In my own eagerness to please her with my approval, I ignored my supervisor's admonition that I was not a literary critic and that to undertake that role would lead me eventually to a choice between dishonesty or hurting her.

One day, well into treatment, she brought a packet of her work. Instead of handing it to me in the usual way, she offhandedly tossed it on a chair. Missing the clues to angry feelings that were already mounting from an earlier slight, I took her gesture to indicate that my opinion was no longer important to her.

In order to demonstrate to her that my opinion still counted, I returned the packet at the next session just as she had presented it, tossing it on the same chair without comment. There followed an outpouring of rage that reverberated for months and nearly brought treatment to a halt.

My attempt to "teach her a lesson" was a dishonest manipulation and a misuse of my power in the relationship. I had ignored the feelings behind my patient's actions and acted out my own unacknowledged feelings toward her.

It is particularly important in treating patients with BPD for therapists continually to monitor their own feelings during treatment. Such awareness will both alert you to potential impasses in treatment and prevent you from acting out feelings in a damaging way. Keeping track of your feelings may also help you decide whether or not an intervention you are considering is appropriate. For example, if you are considering involuntary hospitalization and you are feeling punitive toward your patient, the wisdom of this measure should be carefully reconsidered. Of course, your patient's safety will always be the ultimate deciding factor.

Acknowledge Your Limitations

Even the most skilled therapists are likely to encounter patients they cannot treat. The fit between patient and therapist is an intricate balance. If therapy is not progressing, a change of therapist or treatment setting may be indicated.

If treatment is marked by frequent acting out, such as recurrent suicide attempts or gestures, a closer look at the process is warranted. Your own apprehension about the risk to your patient's life is likely to paralyze your capacity to be therapeutic.

At such times, consultation may be helpful. Since the patient is at risk, an inpatient evaluation may be indicated and referral to a university teaching hospital or a center specializing in treating personality disorders may be an effective use of inpatient resources.

If acting out continues unabated, then ending treatment may be indicated. Discussing this possibility with your patient is an honest acknowledgment of your limitations and may itself break the impasse by confronting her fantasy of your omnipotent capacity to rescue her. Such a discussion would be an appropriate use of your power in the relationship, since your patient's emotional investment in continuing treatment with you may encourage her to control her dangerous behavior.

Many concurrent processes contribute to effective therapy. Some of these are identical to processes occurring in healthy childhood development. One critical element of childhood development is the child's identification with the healthy behaviors modeled by parents. If in the course of therapy, you become a powerless victim, your patient is unlikely to extract herself from the victim role. If, on the other hand, you set effective limits, develop appropriate boundaries, and conduct yourself honestly and responsibly, she is also likely to claim her capacity for self-determination.

Epilogue

As my patients and I sift through the experiences unearthed during therapy, the landscape is littered with debris. Often it is impossible to decide which of the fragments are crucial and which inconsequential to the task. In memories and dreams, the most valuable treasures often appear drab and unobtrusive.

Dreams are rich troves of information that hold more secrets than we can usually discover in a single look. Dreams, in fact, only give up their secrets when the dreamer is emotionally prepared to learn about them. So Sara's dream of being lost in the woods contained most of what she needed to know in order to heal. It could be understood, however, only in the context of the picture that was forming from the other fragments of her experience.

While Sara was drinking, she vented her anger at Lisa, her older child. As Sara's story unfolded, her identification with Lisa became clearer, and we came to understand the intensity of Sara's guilt from her own childhood. Even the timing of her symptoms fit into a logical pattern. Sara first fell ill when Lisa reached the age at which the terror had begun. Her self-punishment occurred for the first time when both girls had reached the ages of Sara and Mark when Mark was first included in the terror. Sara's fantasy that her unborn child had been male was another clue to her lost brother's importance in understanding her pain.

I find most trying in treatment the task of providing safety while at the same time maintaining an alliance with my patient in the exploration we have undertaken. Sara's dwindling weight presented an excruciating dilemma, made even more complex by the uncertainty of the point at which her weight loss would become life-threatening. Since she was unwilling to be rehospitalized, providing her this safety would have brought with it a power struggle. Such decisions involve a judgment call that can easily be wrong.

Not all patients experience the intensity of Sara's turmoil or her close brush with dying. Neither do all patients reach the level of understanding that Sara acquired about the origins of her pain. When we embark upon an expedition, we cannot know whether we will come upon an ancient city, discover a long lost scroll, or spend most of the time sifting through empty sand. We can only hope that something of value will be found that makes the journey worthwhile.

Appendix A
Newer Psychological Treatments

Sit thee down by me, and ease
thine heart in whispers.
JOHN KEATS

For much of the last century, the pillar of psychological treatment for most emotional disorders was psychoanalytic psychotherapy. This approach is based upon psychoanalysis, in which free association is employed to explore thoughts about present-day life, fantasies, dreams, and memories in order to clarify the meaning of symptoms and resolve them. Psychoanalytic psychotherapy involves an ongoing dialogue between patient and therapist, who are mutually engaged in exploring the patient's personal history. The search for the origins of symptoms in past experience was long a basic tenet of all treatment.

This view was challenged with the advent of behavior therapy, which gained prominence in the mid-sixties with the work of Isaac Marks in treating anxiety with exposure therapy. With exposure therapy, patients are confronted, either in imagination or in real life, with situations or memories that have become associated with intense anxiety or other negative emotions. With enough exposure in the absence of actual danger, the intensity of the emotional response dissipates and the situations lose their power.

Combining exposure with relaxation techniques may enhance its effects. Specific behaviors that occur in response to anxiety, such as compulsive washing in response to fears of contamination, can be addressed by preventing the usual response during exposure to an emotionally charged scene. With this combination of exposure and response prevention, both irrational fear and compulsive rituals eventually cease. In this way, dramatic changes in symptoms and behavior can occur without discovering their origins.

Cognitive therapy also addresses symptoms directly by identifying and challenging unrealistic assumptions and beliefs, thereby changing the disturbed emotions and behavior that accompanied them. Cognitive therapy, like behavior therapy, focuses primarily on the here and now. Cognitive and behavioral strategies can be combined, often with rapid and powerful effects upon changing behavior. For example, the assumptions underlying a patient's fear of a situation may be examined and corrected, followed by exposure therapy. Considering the corrected belief while visualizing the situation may further serve to reinforce the new viewpoint.

Interpersonal therapy is a time-limited treatment for depression that focuses on managing current relationships. It deals with the interplay between symptoms and the most important relationships in a patient's life. In interpersonal therapy, the therapist takes an active role in coaching patients to interact more effectively with their spouses and others. Increasing satisfaction in relationships is viewed as a means of increasing emotional well-being and relieving distress.

Psychoanalytic psychotherapy, behavior therapy, cognitive therapy, cognitive-behavior therapy, and interpersonal therapy have all been used to treat various aspects of BPD. Until recently, however, there have been few efforts to design treatments for the specific combination of symptoms that encompass BPD.

Effective treatment for BPD would address all of the following goals:

- Learning to delay impulses, gradually substituting safer and safer behaviors for self-destructive ones.
- Becoming aware of a spectrum of specific emotions, such as sadness, disappointment, loneliness, fear, and anger, instead of just feeling "bad" or "empty."
- Learning to tolerate painful emotions without urgently seeking escape.
- Learning to express feelings verbally, rather than acting them out impulsively. This includes being able to express anger, even toward your therapist.
- Learning to tolerate flaws in yourself and others and still appreciate your fundamental goodness.
- Learning to be alone without feeling lost.
- Developing a stable sense of personal identity with values and beliefs that endure, even when you are hurting.
- Being able to weather momentary misfortune while maintaining hope.

Two novel treatment approaches, Dialectical Behavior Therapy (DBT) and Eye Movement Desensitization and Reprocessing (EMDR), deserve special attention. DBT is a comprehensive program of treatment designed especially to treat BPD. EMDR is a more focused treatment tool designed to treat specific fears and the effects of emotional trauma. While it offers only a partial approach to treating BPD, its strategic integration within a treatment program can produce powerful results.

Dialectical Behavior Therapy

Dialectical Behavior Therapy, developed by Marsha Linehan, Ph.D., at the University of Washington, is the first systematic treatment designed especially to treat Borderline Personality

Disorder. It addresses each of the above treatment goals. It is designed in stages, beginning with teaching patients how to avoid the self-destructive behaviors that threaten their safety and interfere with their ability to engage productively in treatment.

The heart of DBT is seeking balance. People with BPD have had their emotions, perceptions, and behaviors repeatedly invalidated by others throughout their lives. At the same time, they cling desperately to those same familiar ways of dealing with the world that have consistently failed. DBT seeks to restore balance, validating feelings and perceptions by acknowledging their logic within the framework of the patient's experience, while at the same time encouraging change in patterns of behavior that don't work.

DBT is designed to integrate the many separate compartments into which the memories, emotions, and perceptions of people with BPD are divided. The first stage of treatment seeks balance between rational thinking and emotion. It begins by helping patients become more aware or "mindful" of what they are experiencing in the present without judging their feelings or jumping to irrational negative conclusions.

"Mindfulness" means learning to narrate the details of the moment, identifying emotions, the sensory impressions of one's surroundings, and accompanying bodily sensations. Learning to distinguish feelings accurately, such as sadness or disappointment, anger or frustration, terror or foreboding, in place of indescribable misery, can be empowering. Becoming aware of the variety and changing texture of emotions can help momentary pain feel less overwhelming. Observing without judging the nuances of the moment can keep its meaning from becoming exaggerated.

Mindfulness is the foundation upon which patients build skills to regulate emotions. These begin with relaxation and breathing techniques as well as lifestyle changes designed to increase mental acuity and feelings of well-being. It moves on to ways to counter negative emotions and create alternative responses to situations that once triggered self-destructive behaviors. In the beginning, this might mean substituting safer ways to self-inflict pain, such as applying ice cubes to the wrists, in place of more dangerous habits. Later, patients learn constructive ways to self-soothe and become comfortable with nurturing themselves. They may develop creative ways to express emotions through art, poetry, or music. Teaching assertiveness skills is another way that DBT helps patients feel less helpless.

DBT simultaneously seeks to build self-acceptance and self-esteem and to challenge the status quo, relentlessly encouraging changes that will make life more fulfilling. It helps patients find the middle ground between self-condemnation and self-righteousness. The delicate balance between self-acceptance and the relentless pursuit of change is the essential "dialectic" of DBT. Dialectical Behavior Therapy seeks to establish balance in this and other dichotomies of the black-and-white world of BPD.

Once safety measures are in place, broader goals can be addressed. During the middle stage of treatment, the connections between present symptoms and past experience may be explored, using a variety of psychotherapeutic techniques. Traumatic memories might be clarified during a psychoanalytic dialogue and later addressed with exposure techniques to diminish their emotional intensity. Daunting present-day situations might be addressed with exposure and rehearsal of effective new strategies of behavior.

In the final stage of treatment, identity matures, with enduring values and convictions that no longer require validation from others. By this stage, patients have learned that periods of distress are a normal part of living and can be tolerated and survived. Once patients accept that they can feel miserable for a while without having to escape and that they can expect to feel better eventually, they are well on their way to health.

DBT in its complete form includes individual therapy, skills training groups, and real-world interventions. Especially in the earlier stages of treatment, therapists are broadly accessible by telephone to help patients sidetrack self-destructive urges and to coach them through interpersonal crises and other problems as they develop. This goes beyond the usual availability for emergencies that most therapists provide. DBT is therefore more labor-intensive than most other forms of treatment and is ideally provided by a team of clinicians who can both share the task and provide one another support and validation. Many elements of DBT, however, can be adapted for use by individual therapists.

Dr. Linehan and her group have provided training in DBT to therapists all over the world. They have also done systematic outcome studies that indicate that, while DBT is a time-intensive and costly approach to treatment, it brings about a high rate of improvement and reduces the overall cost of medical and psychiatric treatment among patients with BPD.

Eye Movement Desensitization and Reprocessing (EMDR)

Eye Movement Desensitization and Reprocessing, developed by Francine Shapiro, Ph.D., was designed to neutralize the emotional pain accompanying memories of traumatic events. It has been dramatically effective for many patients with Post-Traumatic Stress Disorder, who often suffer from intrusive flashbacks, in which memories of terrifying experiences are vividly recalled as if they were happening in the present. EMDR has ended such waking nightmares for many combat veterans and victims of war, violent crimes, or natural disasters.

Since its inception, EMDR has been applied more broadly to treat symptoms associated with emotional trauma in a variety of disorders. Since many people with BPD have suffered severe abuse, overwhelming loss, or other intensely painful experiences during childhood, EMDR has become an important therapeutic tool in treating this aspect of BPD. It is not intended, however, to be a comprehensive treatment for BPD. How and when it is woven into a treatment approach is crucial to its safety and effectiveness. Because EMDR can evoke powerful emotions, the skills for controlling destructive impulses, such as those taught during the initial stage of Dialectical Behavior Therapy, should be well-developed before EMDR is undertaken.

EMDR combines the simultaneous use of patterned eye movements and imagery in order to rob horrifying memories of their emotional intensity. Most commonly, eye movements are guided by the therapist's hand as it moves rhythmically back and forth across the field of vision while the patient visualizes an emotionally charged scene. EMDR also identifies and seeks to correct negative beliefs about ourselves and the world that have arisen from painful past events and powerfully influence present-day emotions and behavior. While the eye movements are the central feature that distinguishes EMDR from other treatments, EMDR is actually an artful blend of several therapeutic techniques, including exposure therapy, cognitive therapy, and even an abbreviated form of the free association of psychoanalytic psychotherapy.

Memories of intensely distressing events often seem frozen in time, vivid and unchanging in detail long after the actual events have occurred. The emotions accompanying the memories may also remain vivid and feel exactly the same whenever they are recalled. These emotions can be so intense that it feels as if the original threat is still present. Rapid pulse, sweating, chest pain, shortness of breath, and other physical manifestations of fear may accompany them. Such memories may be engraved in the circuitry of the brain so that each episode of recall activates a similar sequence of locations in the brain.

Before an EMDR session is undertaken, a structured interview is performed in which critical elements of the experience to be addressed are defined. A specific memory is selected and the emotions and physical sensations associated with the memory are spelled out in detail. Patients are then asked to identify a present-day negative belief about themselves and the way they experience their lives that seems connected to the memory. They are then asked to construct a positive self-message, however unbelievable it may seem at the time, to replace the negative message. The last stage of an EMDR session involves "installing" or making believable at an emotional level, the positive self-message.

For example, a woman who has been physically abused as a child might identify one or more of the following beliefs about herself that have guided her life:

"I will always be a helpless victim."

"I must always avoid making others angry."

"I deserve to be treated cruelly."

Corresponding corrective positive self-messages might include the following examples:

"I can control my own destiny."

"I have a right to my own opinions."

"I deserve to be happy."

An EMDR session begins with the patient imagining a scene that embodies the essence of a painful situation from the past. The scene is then maintained in awareness while the patient's eyes follow the motion of the therapist's hand. After each set of eye movements, the patient is asked to take a deep breath and then to report briefly whatever is foremost in her awareness. She is then asked to focus on that image, thought, or feeling while going through another set of eye movements. The sequence is repeated until the patient is able to visualize the original scene while remaining completely relaxed. Typical sessions range between 45 and 90 minutes. During the course of a successful EMDR session, both the original scene and any derivative memories lose their emotional intensity.

Once the patient can picture these images while remaining completely relaxed, she is ready to "install" the relevant positive belief. This is accomplished by maintaining simultaneously in awareness the original scene and the positive self-statement while repeating sets of eye movements until the statement feels emotionally valid.

While the above outline may appear deceptively simple, it is only an overview and is not intended to be a guide to technique. Important technical details have been omitted. Moreover, considerable skill and training are required on the therapist's part to guide the process safely and effectively, particularly when emotions become intense or when impasses are reached.

Early theories about EMDR focused on the similarity between its patterned eye movements and the rapid eye movements (REM) that accompany dreaming sleep. Freud called dreams "the royal road to the unconscious." He believed that the content of dreams contained important clues to the dreamer's emotional struggles and became an arena for solving problems and resolving conflict during sleep. More recent theories about the function of REM sleep have placed less emphasis on dream content and more on the physiology of the dreaming state. What is clear is that when deprived of REM sleep, we go to great lengths to replenish it as soon as possible, dreaming more frequently and often more vividly until the deficit has been corrected. From such observations, it has been inferred that the REM stage of sleep is crucial in some way to sleep's restorative function and to emotional health.

Despite the tempting analogy between EMDR and REM sleep, EMDR probably works by a combination of effects. For many people, the eye movements produce a relaxation response, decreasing emotional arousal and the physical symptoms that accompany it. The relaxation response varies considerably both in strength and pace from person to person. This is the "desensitization" part of the treatment.

Moving the eyes also affects the sequence in which different areas of the brain are turned on. For example, moving the eyes back and forth requires sequential activity in both sides of the brain. This patterned activation may replace the rigid patterns associated with the original memory and bring new resources to bear upon how the memory is processed. This in turn would enable the characteristics of the memory, emotions, and accompanying beliefs to change. One consequence of this reprocessing is to allow events to assume their proper place and time in our personal histories, so that they no longer feel current.

I first learned about EMDR and went through training as an EMDR therapist after the original version of *Lost in the Mirror* was completed. It has since become an important part of my therapeutic repertoire. It has helped to overcome impasses that no amount of conventional talking therapy could surmount. With EMDR, patients often discover important connections among experiences and relationships with remarkable speed. What is most impressive is the power of the technique to tap the mind's innate wisdom and creativity. Patients often discover aspects of their experiences that had previously eluded them. These discoveries have been the saving graces that turn tragedy into personal growth.

Candace came to treatment at age 42 because her life had felt completely out of control since an attempted rape at knifepoint seven years previously. She had been severely sexually abused during much of her childhood and had divorced an abusive husband just a year before the attack occurred. When the attacker drove her to a remote wooded area, she was certain that there was no chance of escape and that she would die. She had fought him off, however, managing to kick him hard enough to knock the wind out of him, and had escaped into the woods.

For Candace, the attack was the last straw that convinced her that she would always be a victim. She felt marked for exploitation and helpless to do anything about it. She selected as the starting point for an EMDR session about the attack the moment that she concluded that escape was impossible and that she was going to die. As we began to work, she became immediately in touch with the terror of that scene. As the scene unfolded with successive sets of eye movements, however, she became suddenly aware of the power that enabled her to fight back and to get away. More importantly, she identified that moment as the very first time in her life that she had ever fought back against an aggressor. She had not been raped. And she would no longer regard herself as a helpless victim. At the end of the session, she visualized again the original scene and installed the positive belief, "I am strong and determined."

EMDR can be a powerful and often rapid treatment for trauma. The experience can be intense, however, and may temporarily stir up symptoms. Its power to help carries with it a level of risk in keeping with that power. It should be undertaken only in the hands of a therapist experienced both in EMDR and in treating people with BPD, and only after a trusting therapeutic relationship has been well-established.

Psychotherapy is as much art as science. No single therapeutic technique works equally well for all patients, even if they suffer from similar symptoms. A skilled psychotherapist learns to fit the treatment to the patient and may end up weaving together a variety of approaches over the course of treatment. In the end, the quality of the collaboration between patient and therapist is at least as important as the specific techniques with which they work.

Finally, psychotherapy is not a substitute for biological treatments. Most patients with BPD, even in a highly structured treatment setting, will require medications to help quiet the storm within, at least in the early stages of treatment. Without medication, most patients would be too distracted to engage in the challenging work of psychotherapy. Many will continue to require medication throughout treatment and even after its conclusion. While reducing the need for medication is a worthwhile goal of treatment, a continuing need for it does not diminish the value of a treatment effort that has brought living back to life.

Appendix B
Resources

Since the original publication of *Lost in the Mirror* in 1996, sweeping changes have occurred not only in the information and treatment resources available about BPD, but also in the way that information is disseminated. The Internet has become easily accessible to a growing number of households and provides a wealth of information that is constantly being updated. This edition therefore includes a selection of web sites that I have found particularly informative, including some focused specifically on BPD and related issues and a few mental health sites of general interest. I have selected sites that have track records of at least several years' endurance and which are likely to continue to grow.

In the last five years, there has been a growing public awareness of BPD, with media attention including even a popular movie, *Girl, Interrupted*, that was based on the autobiography of Susannah Kaysen, a woman once treated for the disorder. A number of informative books about BPD have been published that have been written for the benefit of people with BPD and those close to them. Some have been written by professionals and some by survivors of the disorder in various stages of recovery. These new books are now the centerpiece of the reference section. While reference material is still included about the crucial topics of suicide and self-injury, I have not tried in this edition to cover the whole range of related topics, such as dissociative disorders, eating disorders, and abuse.

One tragic turn of events has been the impact of managed care on treatment programs designed to treat BPD and related disorders. Almost all of the programs listed in the first edition have closed. The majority of the programs in a list that I compiled less than a year ago have also closed. A major chain of private psychiatric hospitals filed bankruptcy and recently closed the last of its hospitals, including the one that served my community. It is therefore impossible to provide timely information in a printed publication even on the remaining limited resources. Some of the webmasters of the listed sites are making efforts to keep such information available and current.

While the listings that follow are not exhaustive, they should provide access to an almost bewildering amount of information via references and links. A word of caution should be observed as you seek further information. Some of the readings, particularly those that go into detail about forms of compulsive self-injury, may tend to trigger such urges in some people. If you are being treated for BPD, it would be advisable to ask your therapist to screen such material before you read it.

Organizations

Mental Health and Illness

National Alliance for the Mentally Ill (NAMI). 200 N. Glebe Road, Suite 1015, Arlington, VA 22203-3008. (800) 950-6264 or (750) 524-7600. www.nami.org *Provides referrals to local chapters, which make available information about local resources.*

National Mental Health Association. Mental Health Information Center, 1021 Prince Street, Alexandria VA 22314-2971. (800) 969-6642. www.nmha.org

National Mental Health Consumers Self-Help Clearinghouse. 311 S. Juniper Street, #1000, Philadelphia, PA 19107. (800) 553-4539.

NIMH Public Inquiries, National Institute of Mental Health. 6001 Executive Blvd, Room 8184, MSC 9663, Bethesda, MD 20892-9663. (301) 443-4513. www.nimh.nih.gov e-mail nimhinfo@nih.gov

Self-Injury/Self-Mutilation

S.A.F.E. Alternatives. c/o Karen Conterio and Wendy Lader, Ph.D., 3249 S. Oak Park Avenue, Berwyn, IL 60402. (800) 366-8288. www.SAFE-Alternatives.com

Suicide

American Association of Suicidology. 4201 Connecticut Avenue NW, Suite 408, Washington, DC 20008. (202) 237-2280. www.suicidology.org *Provides information and resources for anyone concerned about suicide, including professionals, people at risk, family members, and survivors.*

American Foundation for Suicide Prevention. 120 Wall Street, Floor 22, New York, NY 10005. (212) 363-3500. www.afsp.org

The Samaritans of USA. 9 Wild Harbor Road, North Falmouth, MA 02556. www.befrienders.org *A part of Befrienders International, a worldwide volunteer organization for suicide prevention. The crisis helplines provide confidential support to anyone in need.*

Web Sites

Befrienders International. www.befrienders.org *A worldwide volunteer organization for suicide prevention. The website includes a directory of crisis helplines and other resources by geographic location.*

Borderline Personality Disorder.
www.palace.net/~llama/psych/bpd.html *Defines BPD from various theoretical perspectives, including those of Kernberg and Gunderson. Included also is an overview of the* Diagnostic Interview for Borderlines, Revised, *a structured diagnostic interview for diagnosing BPD.*

The Borderline Sanctuary. www.mhsanctuary.com/borderline *Recovery information from a number of sources coordinated by Patty Pheil, M.S.W., and her husband Tim Pheil, L.P.N., who have a personal interest in BPD and empathy for its sufferers. An "Ask the Doctor" section features Paul J. Markovitz, M.D., Ph.D., a psychiatrist whose research has focused on biological treatments for BPD.*

Depression Central. www.psycom.net/depression.central.html *A rich source of information on all types of depressive disorders, compiled by psychiatrist Ivan Goldberg, M.D.*

Lifescape.com. www.Lifescape.com *Detailed articles on a variety of mental health conditions and topics, compiled in cooperation with the University of Florida Brain Institute.* Keyword: borderline *will bring up my article on BPD.*

S.A.F.E. Alternatives. www.SAFE-Alternatives.com *This site is dedicated to empowering self-injurers to learn to keep themselves safe. It is maintained by Karen Conterio and Wendy Lader, Ph.D., who run a treatment program for people who self-injure. The site includes information about the program and about a book authored by the program's leaders.*

Self-Help and Psychology Magazine. www.shpm.com *An online magazine featuring original articles covering a wide range of psychological topics of interest both to the general public and to people suffering from specific disorders.*

Self-Injury Resources. www.smalltime.com/notvictims *Valuable information for people who struggle with the compulsion to self-injure.*

Soul's Self-Help Central. www.soulselfhelp.on.ca *An extremely thoughtful and extensive site created by A. J. Mahari, who has recovered from BPD. It contains many useful insights about the recovery process. I have watched both the site and its owner grow considerably over the last several years.*

Further Reading

For Consumers and Professionals

Alderman, Tracy. *The Scarred Soul: Understanding and Ending Self-Inflicted Violence.* Oakland: New Harbinger Publications, 1997. *A compassionate discussion of why people engage in self-inflicted violence, this book also offers concrete exercises to help people stop this behavior. It may also help demystify self-injury for family members and others close to someone who practices it.*

Cauwels, Janice M. *Imbroglio: Rising to the Challenges of Borderline Personality Disorder.* New York: W. W. Norton & Company, 1992. *One of the most ambitious treatises on BPD for the general public, this book, written by a journalist, is drawn from countless interviews with authorities in the field.*

Conterio, Karen, and Wendy Lader. *Bodily Harm: The Breakthrough Healing Program for Self-Injurers.* New York: Hyperion, 1998. *This book discusses self-injury and describes the structured treatment program developed by the authors to help people end it. It provides practical guidelines of use both to people who self-injure and the professionals treating them.*

Kreisman, Jerold J., and Hal Strauss. *I Hate You—Don't Leave Me: Understanding the Borderline Personality.* New York: Avon Books, 1989. *The first and for years the only resource for the non-professional, this book was once considered the "borderline's bible."*

Mason, Paul T., and Randi Kreger. *Stop Walking on Eggshells: Coping When Someone You Care About Has Borderline Personality Disorder.* Oakland: New Harbinger Publications, 1998. *Helpful information and guidance to help anyone in a relationship with someone with BPD weather the storm.*

Miller, Dusty. *Women Who Hurt Themselves: A Book of Hope and Understanding*. New York: Basic Books, 1994. *This book provides a framework for understanding self-harm and self-inflicted pain as reenactment of early traumatic experiences.*

Santoro, Joseph. *The Angry Heart: Overcoming Borderline and Addictive Disorders*. Oakland: New Harbinger Publications, 1997. *Written partly in the autobiographical voice of the fictional Samuel, this book presents information about BPD and the treatment approach developed by its author, a clinical psychologist.*

Shapiro, Francine, and Margot S. Forrest. *EMDR: The Breakthrough Therapy for Overcoming Anxiety, Stress, and Trauma*. New York: Basic Books, 1997. *Co-authored by the psychologist who developed EMDR, this book is a helpful introduction to the treatment for anyone contemplating undergoing it.*

Thornton, Melissa F. *Eclipses: Behind the Borderline Personality Disorder*. Madison, AL: Monte Sano Publishing, 1997. *Written by a person recovering from BPD, this book presents an engaging and informative account of what it is like to experience treatment with Dialectical Behavior Therapy in an inpatient setting.*

Primarily for Professionals

Favazza, Armando R. *Bodies Under Siege: Self-Mutilation and Body Modification in Culture and Society*. Second Edition. Baltimore: Johns Hopkins University Press, 1996.

Gunderson, John G. *Borderline Personality Disorder*. Washington: American Psychiatric Press, 1984.

Kernberg, Otto. *Borderline Conditions and Pathological Narcissism*. New York: Jason Aronson, 1975.

Kernberg, Otto, and Michael A. Seltzer, et al. *Psychodynamic Psychotherapy of Borderline Patients*. New York: Basic Books, 1989.

Kroll, Jerome. *PTSD-Borderlines in Therapy: Finding the Balance*. New York: W. W. Norton & Company, 1993.

Linehan, Marsha M. *Cognitive-Behavioral Treatment of Borderline Personality Disorder*. New York: The Guilford Press, 1993.

————. *Skills Training Manual for Treating Borderline Personality Disorder.* New York: The Guilford Press, 1993.

Masterson, James F. *The Narcissistic and Borderline Disorders: An Integrated Developmental Approach.* New York: Brunner/Mazel, 1981.

Paris, Joel M. *Borderline Personality Disorder: A Multidimensional Approach.* Washington: American Psychiatric Press, 1994.

Stone, Michael A. *The Fate of Borderline Patients: Successful Outcome and Psychiatric Practice.* New York: The Guilford Press, 1990.

Strong, Marilee. *A Bright Red Scream: Self-Mutilation and the Language of Pain.* New York: Penguin, 1999.

To Enrich the Soul

Albom, Mitch. *Tuesdays with Morrie: An Old Man, a Young Man, and Life's Greatest Lesson.* New York: Doubleday, 1997. *The most recent addition to a timeless list, this book is about love, friendship, and savoring life on whatever terms it offers.*

Buscaglia, Leo F. *Loving Each Other: The Challenge of Human Relationships.* New York: Fawcett Books, 1990.

Carroll, Lewis. *Journeys in Wonderland.* New York: Derrydale Books, 1979.

Frankl, Victor E. *Man's Search for Meaning.* New York: Washington Square Press, 1998.

Kushner, Harold S. *When Bad Things Happen to Good People.* New York: Avon Books, 1994.

Rubin, Theodore I. *Compassion and Self-Hate: An Alternative to Despair.* New York: Touchstone, 1998.

Viorst, Judith. *Necessary Losses.* New York: Fireside, 1998.

Williams, Margery. *The Velveteen Rabbit.* New York: Simon & Schuster, 1983.

Index

A

Abandonment, 7
  threat of, 144
Abstinence, 126–27
Abuse, 32
  acts of, 45
  alcohol, 7, 45–46, 67–68, 126, 138, 166
  emotional, 39, 152
  physical, 14, 21, 31, 39, 50, 58
  self-, 60, 64
  sexual, 14, 31, 39, 42–43, 44, 50, 52, 58, 152, 167
  substance, 7, 64, 67–68, 126, 138, 166
  in therapy, 88–89
Addiction
  physical, 119
  psychological, 119
Affective (emotional) instability, 9
After-hours calls to therapist, 92
Aggression, 64. *See also* Anger
  controlled, 136
  working out, 33–34
Aging, 57
Agranulocytosis, 118
Alcohol, 34
  abuse of, 7, 45–46, 67–68, 126, 138, 166
Alcohol dependence, case study in, 19–20
Alcoholics Anonymous (AA), 84, 128

Alcoholism, 33
  Korsakoff's Psychosis and, 24–25
Alprazolam (Xanax), 119–20, 120
American Association of Suicidology, 193
American Foundation for Suicide Prevention, 193
Amitriptyline (Elavil), 112, 113
Amnesia, 45
Anger, 7, 34, 135–41. *See also* Aggression
  handling of, 13
  inappropriate, 9
  intense, 9
  as trigger for drinking, 137–38
Anorexia nervosa, 65, 129
  case study in, 19
Antidepressants, 112–16
Antipsychotic drugs, 117–19
Antisocial Personality Disorder, 34
Anxiety, 9, 120
Assertive expression of feelings, 137
Atonement, 65
Attitudes, paradox in, 15
Audiotaped messages, 130

B

Befrienders International, 194
Behavior cluster, 8